GUT HEALTH DIET COOKBOOK

A Practical and Healthy Approach to Eating for Your Gut with Lots of Gut-Friendly Recipes including a 2-Week Meal Plan and Targeted Exercises to Strengthen Your Gut and Promote Your Digestive Health.

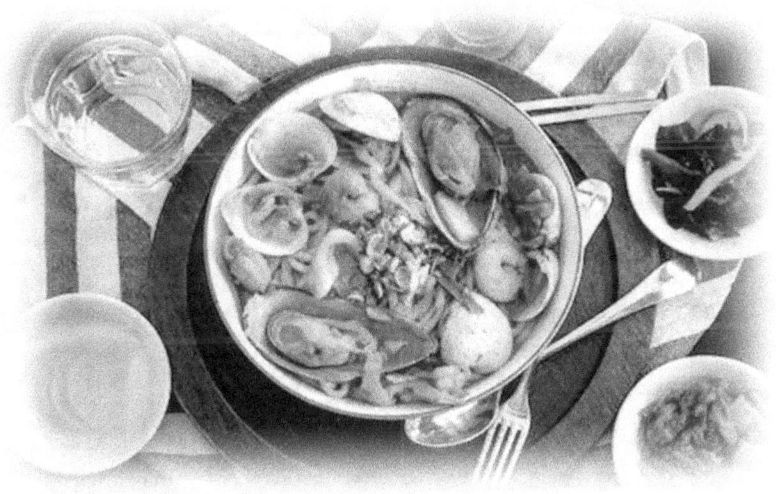

Christiana White

GAIN ACCESS TO MORE BOOKS

TABLE OF CONTENTS.

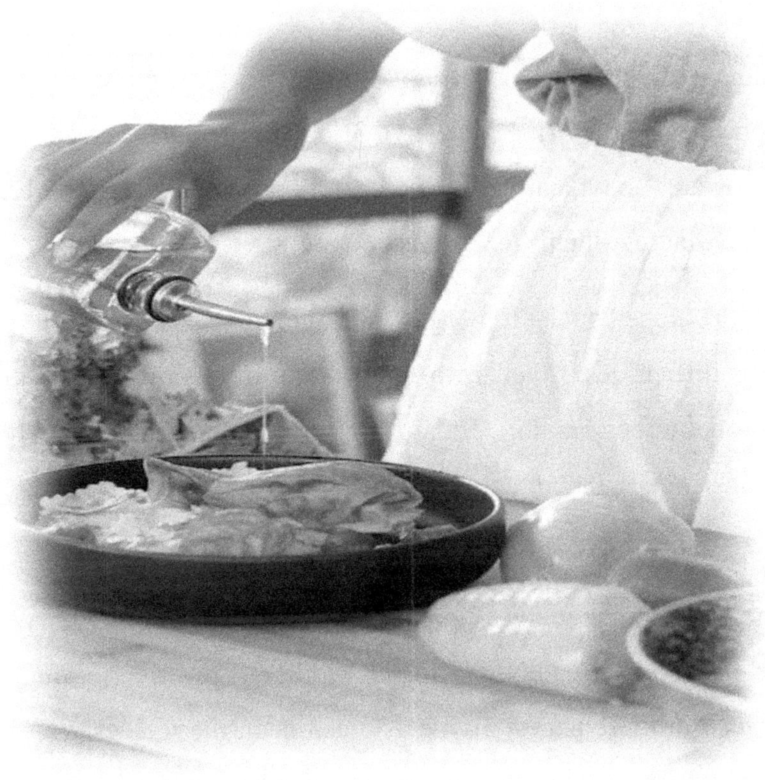

INTRODUCTION

In the quiet corners of kitchens, where sizzling pans and the perfume of fresh herbs coexist, a culinary revolution is taking place—one that goes beyond flavor and into the domain of intestinal health. Welcome to the Gut Health Diet Cookbook, a transforming handbook that has already affected many people's lives, providing solace and empowerment to those struggling with gut health difficulties.

Sarah, a lively lady in her thirties who was previously limited by the discomfort of recurring digestive problems, found herself at a crossroads. The typical paths of comfort appeared elusive until she wandered across the pages of this cookbook.

Sarah developed a way to not just manage, but prevail over her gut health difficulties, thanks to delectable dishes and insightful nutritional understanding. Today, she exudes Vigor, demonstrating the transformational potential of conscious eating.

Then there's Mark, a seasoned adventurer whose global travels were previously hampered by unpredictable intestinal problems. With some hesitation, he delved into the world of gut-friendly cuisine described in these pages. To his astonishment, the recipes not only served as a passport to gastronomic delight, but also revealed a newfound resilience, allowing him to completely embrace life's adventures without reservation.

This is more than simply a recipe; it is a source of hope for individuals traversing the complicated terrain of gut health issues. Whether you want to stop bloating, get rid of indigestion, or take a more holistic approach to your health, this book is for you.

You might wonder what distinguishes this cookbook from the multitude of wellness guides. The answer lies in its combination of delicious meals, evidence-based nutritional insights, and a dedication to promoting long-term well-being. It goes beyond the typical prescriptions, providing a tapestry of Flavors that not only nourish the body but also satisfy the soul.

Imagine the pleasure of enjoying a delectable Probiotic-Rich Roast Chicken that not only tantalizes your taste buds but also feeds the billions of microorganisms in your stomach. Consider the comfort of a Healing Chicken Soup, its warmth embracing you on a cold night while actively supporting your digestive health.

This cookbook is more than just a compilation of recipes; it's a guide to a healthier relationship with food—one that prioritizes intestinal health without sacrificing gastronomic delight. It's a guide that will help you reclaim control of your health by delivering more than just recipes but also a holistic approach to living a thriving life.

So come with us on this journey of flavor, healing, and empowerment.

The Gut Health Diet Cookbook is more than simply a book; it's a guide, a confidant, and a catalyst for transformational change. It's time to enjoy a life in which your gut health thrives and each meal is a step toward wellness. Take the first bite, and the trip begins.

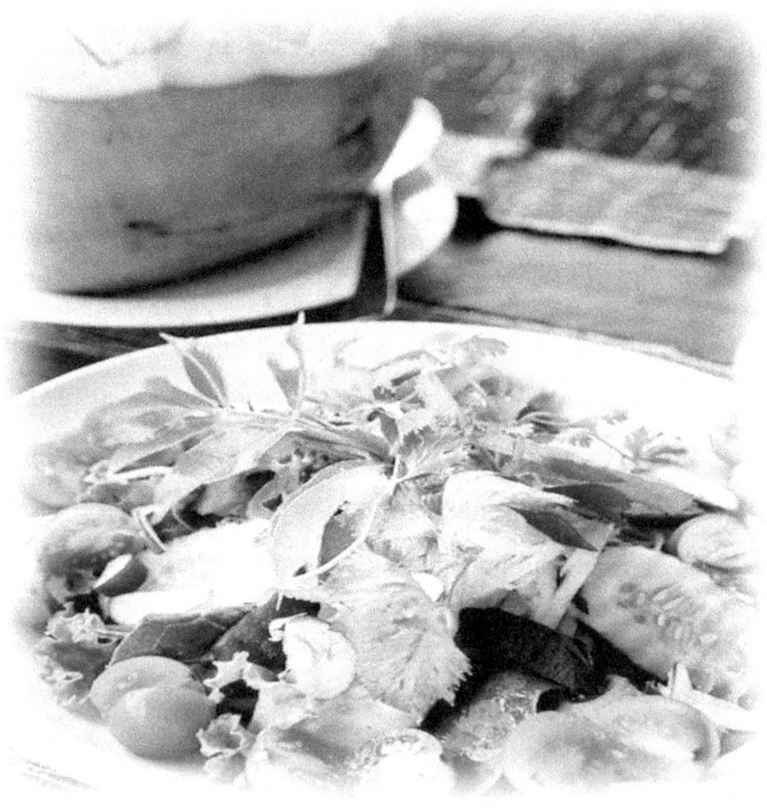

CHAPTER 1

The Significance of Gut Health

Gut health refers to the digestive system's overall health, which influences mood, immunity, and other factors. Your body contains trillions of bacteria, viruses, and fungus, together known as the microbiome. The majority of them live in your intestines, where they help with digestion, immunity, and weight regulation.

The gut microbiome affects your body from the moment you are born, and its composition and diversity are influenced by a variety of factors including genetics, nutrition, lifestyle, drugs, and environmental exposures. A healthy gut has a wide variety of microorganisms, each with particular nutritional preferences and functions.

However, an imbalanced or disrupted gut flora can cause or contribute to a variety of gut-related and systemic illnesses, including IBS, IBD, obesity, diabetes, melancholy, and anxiety. As a result, having a healthy gut is critical for your overall health.

Gut Microbiome and General Well-Being

The gut microbiome communicates with the rest of the body, particularly the brain, via the gut-brain axis, which influences mood, cognition, and behaviour. The gut microbiota also influences the immune system's susceptibility and reaction to infections, allergies, and autoimmune illnesses. Furthermore, the gut flora effects your metabolism, including weight, blood sugar, cholesterol, and blood pressure.

Improving your gut flora can benefit your general well-being by lowering stress, improving sleep, increasing energy, and fostering happiness. Animal models, human research, and question-and-answer sessions have all contributed to an increasing body of evidence linking the gut microbiota to human health.

Principles of Gut-Friendly Diets

A gut-friendly diet promotes the balance and diversity of beneficial bacteria in your stomach. Most people adhere to certain general concepts, such as:

- **Consuming a diverse selection of plant-based foods**, including fruits, vegetables, whole grains, nuts, seeds, and legumes. These foods contain fiber, which feeds beneficial bacteria and creates short-chain fatty acids with anti-inflammatory and immune-boosting properties.

- **Consuming fermented foods** such as yogurt, kefir, sauerkraut, kimchi, and kombucha, which contain live probiotics that colonize and improve gut health.
- **Avoiding or limiting processed foods**, refined sugars, artificial sweeteners, alcohol, and antibiotics, as they can disturb the gut flora and lead to inflammation, leaky gut, and dysbiosis.
- **Selecting organic and grass-fed animal products** that are devoid of hormones, antibiotics, and pesticides, which can disrupt the gut microbiome and raise the risk of chronic diseases.
- **Drinking plenty of water and herbal teas** to hydrate, cleanse, and strengthen the gut mucosal barrier.

A gut-friendly diet might vary according to your own needs, tastes, and goals. You can experiment with different foods to see how they impact your gut health and symptoms. For further personalized advice and guidance, consult a qualified dietitian or nutritionist.

CHAPTER 2

Gut-Friendly Ingredients

One of the keys to maintaining a healthy gut is to eat foods that support helpful bacteria in your digestive tract while inhibiting the growth of dangerous microorganisms. These foods, known as gut-friendly nutrients, contain probiotics, prebiotics, fiber, and some herbs and spices. Here are some examples of each category and how they can help with gut health.

Probiotic-Rich Foods

Probiotics are live microorganisms that colonize the gut and provide a variety of health benefits, including improved digestion, increased immunity, and infection prevention. Fermented foods include probiotics, including yogurt, kefir, sauerkraut, kimchi, kombucha, and miso.

These foods are fermented by bacteria or yeast, resulting in the production of lactic acid, alcohol, or other substances that preserve the food while also improving its flavor and texture.

Probiotic-rich meals can improve the diversity and balance of your gut microbiota, which is the population of bacteria that live in your intestines. A healthy gut microbiome is linked to a lower risk of obesity, diabetes, inflammatory bowel disease, and mental disorders. Probiotics can also assist to regulate your immune system, reduce inflammation, and generate vitamins and short-chain fatty acids that are good for your metabolism and intestinal health.

To get the most out of probiotic-rich foods, eat them on a daily basis and select items with live and active cultures.

You should also avoid pasteurized, heated, or cooked foods, as these processes can destroy the probiotics. Furthermore, seek for products that contain a variety of probiotic strains, as each strain may have a different effect on your gut health.

Fiber-Rich Vegetables, Fruits, And Whole Grains

Fiber is a carbohydrate that your body cannot digest, but intestinal microorganisms can. Fiber is categorized into two types: soluble and insoluble. Soluble fiber dissolves in water and produces a gel-like substance in the gut, slowing digestion, lowering cholesterol, and regulating blood sugar levels. Insoluble fiber does not dissolve in water and adds volume to your stool, preventing constipation and increasing bowel movements.

Fiber-rich foods, such as vegetables, fruits, and whole grains, help nourish your gut flora and promote their growth and activity. This can lead to the formation of beneficial compounds including short-chain fatty acids, which nourish intestinal cells, reduce inflammation, and protect against colon cancer. Fiber can also help prevent the formation of dangerous bacteria, which can lead to infections, inflammation, and dysbiosis.

According to the Academy of Nutrition and Dietetics, you should consume at least 25 grams of fiber per day for women and 38 grams for men.

You should also consume a range of fiber sources, as different forms of fiber might have varied effects on your gut health. Beans, lentils, berries, apples, pears, oats, quinoa, barley, and bran are among the highest-fiber foods.

Herbs & Spices with Digestive Benefits

Herbs and spices not only add flavor to your food, but they can help improve your intestinal health. Many herbs and spices have anti-inflammatory, antioxidant, antibacterial, and carminative qualities that can help reduce intestinal inflammation, scavenge free radicals, slow the growth of dangerous bacteria, and avoid gas and bloating. Some of the best herbs and spices for your gut are:

• **Turmeric**: This brilliant yellow spice includes curcumin, a substance with strong anti-inflammatory and antioxidant properties. Turmeric helps reduce inflammation in the gut, protect against ulcerative colitis, and prevent colon cancer. Turmeric can also boost bile production, which helps with fat digestion and absorption.

• **Ginger**: This spicy root has been used for millennia to cure a variety of digestive issues, including nausea, vomiting, indigestion, and diarrhea. Ginger can increase saliva and stomach secretions, which aids digestion and motility.

Ginger can also calm intestinal muscles, reducing cramps and spasms. Ginger can also prevent the formation of Helicobacter pylori, a bacterium that causes stomach ulcers and gastritis.

• **Cinnamon**: This sweet and aromatic spice can aid with blood sugar regulation, which can impact gut health and hunger. Cinnamon can also boost digestive enzyme activity, resulting in better nutrient digestion and absorption.

Cinnamon can also have antibacterial and antifungal properties, which can help prevent infections and candida buildup in the gut.

• **Peppermint**: This pleasant plant can alleviate a variety of digestive issues, including indigestion, gas, bloating, and IBS. Peppermint can relax the smooth muscles of the intestines, reducing spasms and pain. Peppermint can help increase bile flow, which aids fat digestion and absorption. Peppermint can also have antibacterial and antiviral properties that can help prevent infections and inflammation in the gut.

• **Fennel**: This crisp, bacterium vegetable helps aid digestion and reduce gas and bloating. Fennel can increase stomach secretions, which improves digestion and motility. Fennel can also calm intestinal muscles, reducing cramps and spasms. Fennel can also have antibacterial and antifungal properties, which can help prevent infections and candida buildup in the gut.

Understanding Nutrients and Gut Health

Aside from probiotics, prebiotics, fiber, and herbs & spices, other nutrients are required to maintain a healthy gut. These nutrients include vitamins, minerals, antioxidants, and omega-3 fatty acids, which can support many elements of your gut health, such as:

• **Zinc**: Zinc is a trace mineral that participates in numerous enzymatic activities in the body, including those related to digestion and immunity. Zinc can help keep the gut lining intact, hence preventing leaky gut syndrome and food intolerances.

Zinc can also help regulate stomach acid production, which is required for proper digestion and protection against infections. Zinc can also influence the immune system, lowering inflammation and infection in the stomach. Oysters, red meat, poultry, dairy, eggs, legumes, nuts, and seeds are excellent sources of zinc.

• **Magnesium**: Magnesium is a mineral that affects over 300 metabolic activities in the body, including muscle and neuron function, energy production, and blood pressure management. Magnesium can help relax the muscles of the gut, improving digestion and preventing constipation.

Magnesium can also assist regulate electrolytes in the body, affecting fluid balance and intestinal hydration. Magnesium can also have anti-inflammatory and antioxidant properties, thereby protecting the gut from oxidative stress and damage. Spinach, avocado, anchovies, and dark chocolate are excellent sources of magnesium.

• **Vitamin D**: Vitamin D, a fat-soluble vitamin, is mostly produced by the skin when exposed to sunshine. Vitamin D can control calcium and phosphorus intake, both of which are necessary for bone health and muscle contraction.

Vitamin D can also alter the immune system, influencing inflammation and infections in the gut. Vitamin D can also influence the composition and variety of gut bacteria, affecting gut metabolism and immunity. Fatty fish, egg yolks, mushrooms, and fortified meals are excellent sources of vitamin D.

• **Vitamin C:** This water-soluble vitamin is well-known for its involvement in immunity, wound healing, and collagen synthesis. Vitamin C can also promote gut health by functioning as an antioxidant, scavenging free radicals and protecting the gut from oxidative stress and damage.

Vitamin C can also help with iron absorption, which is required for red blood cell synthesis and oxygen delivery to the gut. Vitamin C can also assist regulate the immune system, reducing inflammation and infections in the stomach. Citrus fruits, berries, peppers, broccoli, and kiwi are excellent sources of vitamin C.

• **Omega-3 fatty acids** are polyunsaturated fatty acids with anti-inflammatory and cardioprotective properties. Omega-3 fatty acids can help lower gastrointestinal inflammation, thereby preventing or treating illnesses including inflammatory bowel disease, ulcerative colitis, and Crohn's disease.

Omega-3 fatty acids can also assist regulate the immune system, reducing inflammation and infections in the stomach. Omega-3 fatty acids can potentially influence the composition and variety of the gut microbiota, hence affecting gut metabolism and immunity.

Fatty fish, flaxseeds, chia seeds, walnuts, and algae are excellent sources of omega-3 fatty acids.

CHAPTER 3

Breakfast

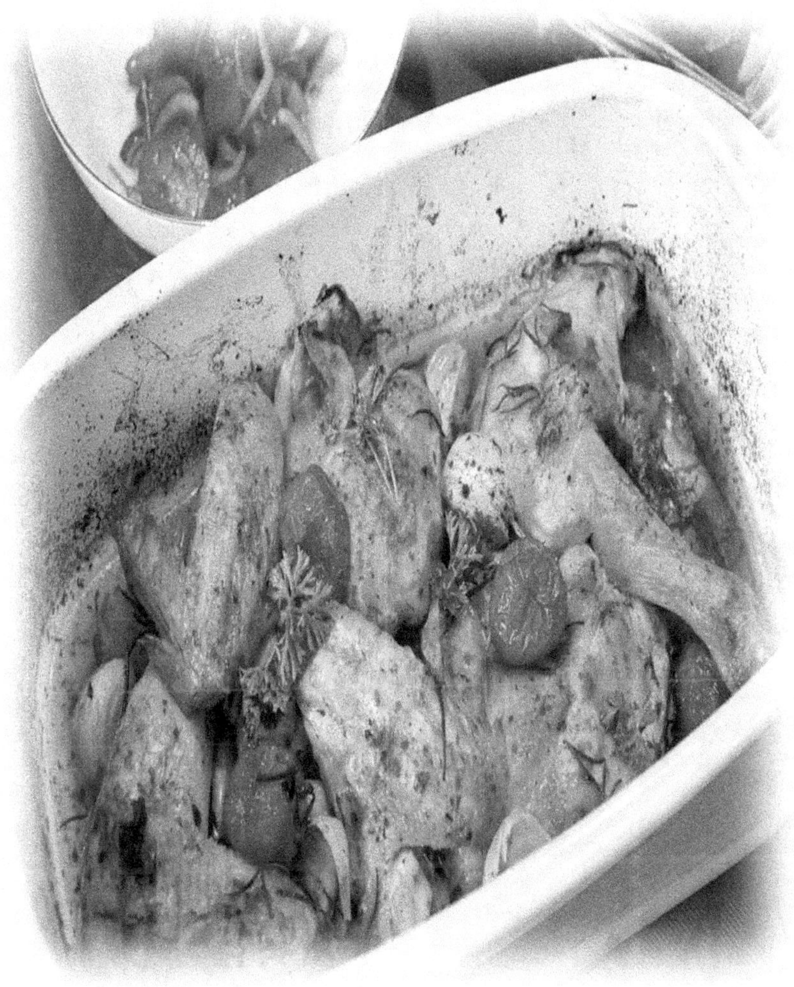

Kefir, Banana, Almond, And Frozen Berry Smoothie.

- *Servings: two.*
- *Prepare time: 5 minutes.*

Ingredients:

- One ripe banana.
- 350 mL kefir
- 75g frozen mixed berries.
- 40-gram whole almonds
- One tablespoon maple syrup or runny honey.

Step-by-step Directions:

- Place everything in a blender or food processor and process until perfectly smooth.
- Pour into two glasses, and serve.

Spring Green Shakshuka

- *Serves: 2-3.*

- *Prepare time: 30 minutes.*

Ingredients:

- Twelve asparagus tips.

- 100 g peas.

- 100g of double-podded broad beans.

- 200 g spinach, shredded

- Olive oil.

- Butter.

- 6 baby leeks (sliced)

- 2 garlic cloves, sliced

- 2 teaspoons cumin seeds.

- 4-6 eggs

- A handful of dill, chopped

- A sprinkling of chilli flakes (optional)

Step-by-step Directions:

- Bring a pan of salted water to a boil, then add the asparagus. Cook for 30 seconds. Add the peas and beans and boil for another 30 seconds, then add the spinach and simmer for 2 seconds longer before draining everything in a sieve.

- Heat 2 tablespoons olive oil and a knob butter in a big frying pan. Cook the leeks and garlic until softened, then add the cumin seeds.
- Stir in the blanched vegetables and simmer for 3-4 minutes. Season, then poke holes for as many eggs as you like and crack an egg into each one.
- Cook gently on the hob until the eggs are cooked to your liking (cover with a lid to hurry things up). Before serving, sprinkle dill and chili flakes over top and drizzle with more olive oil.

Vegan Overnight Oats

- *Serves: 1*
- *Preparation time: 5 minutes plus overnight soak.*

Ingredients:

- 1/2 cup rolled oats.
- 1 cup plant-based milk of your preference
- One tablespoon of chia seeds.
- 1 teaspoon of vanilla extract.
- 1 tablespoon maple syrup or another sweetener (optional)
- Toppings of your choice, such as fresh or dried fruits, nuts, seeds, or coconut flakes.

Step-by-step Directions:

- In a jar or bowl, combine the oats, milk, chia seeds, vanilla, and sweetener, if desired. Stir well, then cover with a lid or plastic wrap.
- Refrigerate overnight or for at least four hours.
- Stir the oats in the morning, adding more milk as needed to achieve the desired consistency.
- Add your toppings and eat cold, or warm up in the microwave if you like.

Figs On Toast with Goat Yogurt Labneh.

- **Servings: six.**
- **Prep time: 15 minutes, with overnight hanging.**

Ingredients:

- 250ml goat's yogurt blended with ¼ tsp salt.
- A few sprigs of thyme and selected leaves
- Six slices of sourdough
- 4-6 ripe figs (sliced)
- Runny honey to serve.

Step-by-step Directions:

- To create the labneh, line a sieve with muslin or a clean J-cloth and add the salted yogurt.
- Place the sieve over a bowl, cover with clingfilm, and store in the refrigerator overnight.
- When ready to serve, transfer the labneh to a bowl and whisk with the thyme.
- Spread the labneh generously on the toast. Top with figs, honey, and a few more thyme leaves.

Miso Chickpeas with Avocado on Toast.

• Servings: two.

• Prepare time: 15 minutes.

Ingredients:

- 400g chickpeas (drained and washed)
- One tablespoon of white miso paste.
- One teaspoon of toasted sesame oil
- 1 lemon, ½ juiced and wedges for serving
- One large avocado.
- 4 small crusty wholemeal or rye bread slices, thick and toasted
- A sprinkle of sesame seeds

- One spring onion, thinly sliced diagonally.

Step-by-Step Directions:

- Combine the chickpeas, miso, sesame oil, lemon juice, and spices in a bowl. Use a potato masher to combine everything until you have a rough paste.
- Transfer the avocado to another basin and mash with a fork until roughly crushed.
- Fold the avocado into the chickpeas and spread over the toast.
- Garnish with sesame seeds and chopped spring onions. Serve with lemon wedges to squeeze over.

Healthy Banana Pancakes

- *Servings: two.*
- *Prepare time: 15 minutes.*

Ingredients:

- Two ripe bananas.
- 2 eggs
- 1/4 cup of whole wheat flour.
- 1/4 teaspoon baking powder.
- 1/4 teaspoon cinnamon.
- Cooking spray or oil.

- Your choice of toppings, such as maple syrup, fresh berries, nut butter, etc.

Step-by-step Directions:

- Using a large bowl, mash the bananas until smooth. Add the eggs and whisk until thoroughly mixed.
- Mix in the flour, baking powder, and cinnamon until you have a thick batter.
- Preheat a large nonstick skillet over medium heat and gently coat with cooking spray or oil. Drop about 1/4 cup batter per pancake onto the skillet and cook for 2-3 minutes, or until bubbles appear on the surface.
- Flip and heat for an additional 1-2 minutes, or until golden and cooked through.
- Repeat with the remaining batter, adding extra oil or spray as needed.
- Top the pancakes with your favorite toppings and enjoy

Raspberry, Peach, And Mango Smoothie Bowl

- *Serves: 1*
- *Prep time is 10 minutes.*

Ingredients:

- One cup of frozen mango chunks.
- 3/4 cup non-fat plain Greek yogurt.
- 1/4 cup of reduced-fat milk.
- 1 teaspoon of vanilla extract.
- 1/4 ripe peach, sliced
- One-third cup raspberries
- 1 tbsp sliced almonds, roasted as desired
- 1 tbsp unsweetened coconut flakes, toasted as desired.
- One teaspoon of chia seeds

Step-by-step Directions:

- In a blender, combine mangos, yogurt, milk, and vanilla. Puree till smooth.
- Pour the smoothie into a bowl and top with peach slices, raspberries, almonds, coconut, and chia seeds as desired.

White Bean and Avocado Toast.

- *Serves: 1*
- *Prep time is 10 minutes.*

Ingredients:

- Toast one slice of whole wheat bread.
- 1/4 avocado, mashed
- Rinse and drain 1/2 cup canned white beans.
- Add kosher salt to taste.
- Grind pepper to taste.
- One pinch of crushed red pepper.

Step-by-step Directions:

- In a small bowl, mash the beans with a fork until they are slightly chunky. Season with salt, pepper, and crushed red pepper as desired.
- Spread mashed avocado on the toast. Top with the bean mixture and enjoy.

Berry-Kefir Smoothie

- *Serves: 1*
- *Prepare time: 5 minutes.*

Ingredients:

- 1-1/2 cups frozen mixed berries
- One cup plain kefir.
- 1/2 medium banana.
- 2 teaspoons almond butter.
- 1/2 teaspoon vanilla extract.

Step-by-step Directions:

- In a blender, combine the berries, kefir, banana, almond butter, and vanilla. Blend until smooth.
- Pour into a large glass or mason jar and enjoy!

Chocolate Banana Oatmeal.

- **Serves: 1**
- **Prep time is 10 minutes.**

Ingredients:

- One cup of water.
- A pinch of salt.
- Half cup old-fashioned rolled oats
- 1/2 small banana, cut
- One tablespoon of chocolate-hazelnut spread.
- Pinch flaky sea salt.

Step-by-step Directions:

- In a small saucepan, heat water and a pinch of normal salt till boiling.
- Stir in the oats, decrease the heat to medium, and simmer, stirring periodically, until the liquid has been absorbed, about 5 minutes. Remove from heat, cover, and allow stand for 2 to 3 minutes.
- Top with bananas, chocolate spread, and flaky salt.

CHAPTER 4

Beef And Pork.

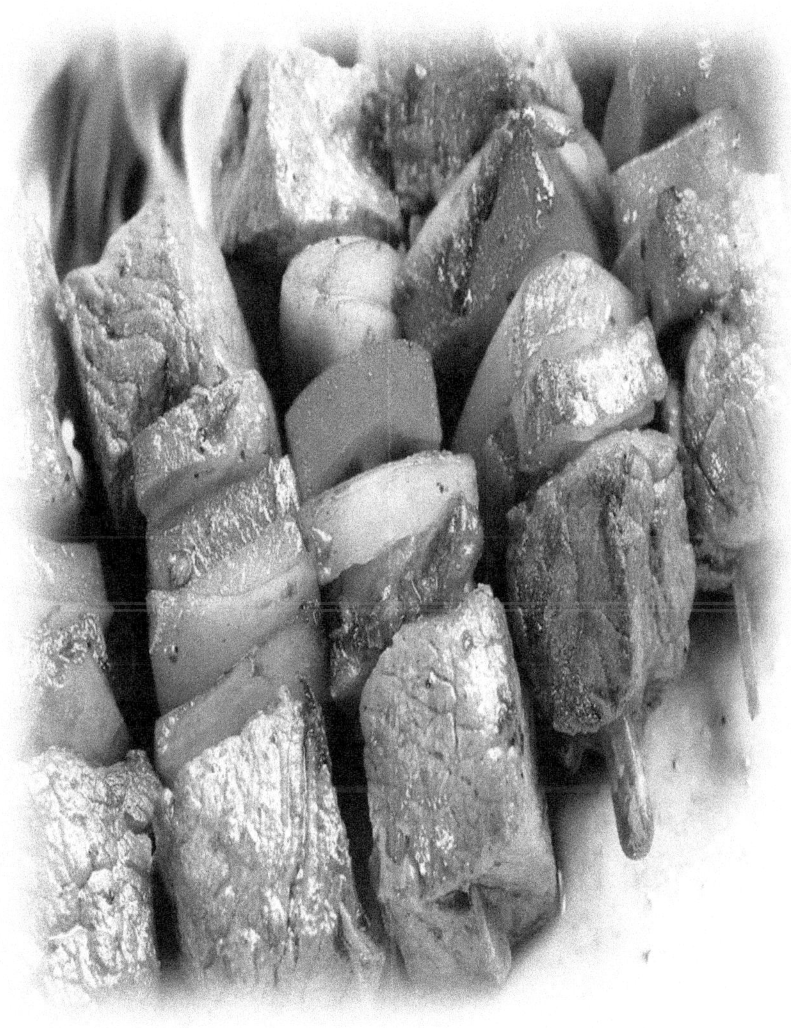

<u>*Cassoulet Recipe.*</u>

- *Serves: 8*
- *Prep time is 20 minutes.*
- *Cooking time: 6 hours on low, 3 hours on high (slow cooker), or 2 hours (Dutch oven).*

Ingredients

- One tablespoon of olive oil.
- Cut 1 pound of pork tenderloin into 1-inch slices.
- Salt and pepper to taste.
- 8 bone-in, skinless chicken thighs (about 2 lbs)
- 8 ounces sliced turkey sausage.
- One large onion, chopped
- 4 garlic cloves, minced
- Two teaspoons dried thyme.
- Two teaspoons of dried rosemary.
- Two bay leaves.
- 4 cups of reduced sodium chicken broth.
- Two (15-ounce) cans of drained and washed white beans.
- 2 big peeled and sliced carrots.
- Two celery stalks, cut
- 1/4 cup chopped fresh parsley.
- Two teaspoons of cornstarch.
- One-quarter cup water

Step-by-step instructions.

- Preheat the oil in a large skillet over medium-high heat. Season the pork with salt and pepper, then brown on all sides for about 10 minutes. Transfer to a large Dutch oven or 6-quart slow cooker.

- In the same skillet, brown the chicken thighs on both sides for about 15 minutes. Transfer to the slow cooker or Dutch oven with the sausage.

- Cook the onion and garlic in the same skillet over medium heat, turning periodically, until softened, about 10 minutes. Bring the thyme, rosemary, bay leaves, and broth to a boil. Pour the beef and beans into the slow cooker or Dutch oven.

- If using a slow cooker, cover and cook on low for 6 hours or high for 3 hours, until the meat is cooked.

- If using a Dutch oven, bring to a boil, then reduce to a simmer and cover for about 2 hours, or until the meat is cooked.

- In a small mixing basin, combine the cornstarch and water. Whisk until smooth. Stir into the cassoulet and cook until slightly thickened, about 15 minutes, on high (slow cooker) or medium-high (Dutch oven).

- Stir in the parsley and season with salt and pepper as needed. Enjoy!

Bratwurst And Sauerkraut.

- *Servings: four.*
- *Prep time is 10 minutes.*
- *Cook for 20 minutes.*

Ingredients

- Four bratwurst sausages.
- Two tablespoons of butter.
- One large onion, sliced
- Two teaspoons of caraway seeds.
- 4 cups of sauerkraut (drained and washed)
- One-quarter cup apple cider vinegar
- Two teaspoons of brown sugar.
- Salt and pepper to taste.
- 4 whole wheat buns, toasted
- Mustard (for serving)

Step-by-step instructions.

- Pierce the sausages all over with a fork. Cook the sausages in a large skillet over medium-high heat, rotating regularly, until they are browned and cooked through, about 15 minutes. Transfer to a dish to keep heated.

- In the same skillet, melt the butter over medium heat. Cook the onion and caraway seeds, stirring periodically, until tender and golden, about 15 minutes.

- Bring the sauerkraut, vinegar, and brown sugar to a boil.

- Reduce the heat to a simmer and stir occasionally for about 10 minutes, or until the liquid has been reduced. Season with salt and pepper to taste.

- Place the sausages on the buns and top with the sauerkraut mixture and mustard. Enjoy!

Jägerschnitzel (Pork Schnitzel with Mushroom Gravy)

- *Servings: four.*
- *Prep time is 20 minutes.*
- *Cook for 20 minutes.*

Ingredients

- Four pork cutlets, pressed thin

- Salt and pepper to taste.

- 1/4 cup all-purpose flour.

- Two eggs, beaten

- 1 cup of breadcrumbs.

- Four teaspoons of vegetable oil.

- Two tablespoons of butter.

- 1 onion, chopped

- Eight ounces of chopped mushrooms

- Two teaspoons of flour.

- Two cups of beef broth.

- Two tablespoons of sour cream.

- 2 tablespoons Worcestershire sauce.

- 2 tablespoons Dijon mustard.

- 2 teaspoons of freshly chopped parsley.

Step-by-step instructions

- Sprinkle the pork cutlets with salt and pepper on both sides. Coat them with flour, shaking off any excess, then dip them in beaten eggs before coating with bread crumbs and pressing to adhere.

- Preheat the oil in a large skillet over medium-high heat. Fry the cutlets in batches until golden and crisp, about 3 minutes each side. Place on a dish and keep warm in the oven.

- In the same skillet, melt the butter over medium heat. Cook the onion and mushrooms, stirring occasionally, until soft and browned, about 15 minutes.

- Sprinkle the flour over the onion and mushroom combination and whisk for 1 minute.

- Gradually whisk in the broth, scraping away any browned pieces from the pan bottom. Bring to a boil, then reduce to a simmer, stirring until slightly thickened, about 10 minutes.

- Add the sour cream, Worcestershire sauce, mustard, and parsley. Season with salt and pepper to taste.

- Serve the pork cutlets with mushroom gravy and enjoy.

French Dip Sandwich

- *Servings: four.*
- *Prep time is 10 minutes.*
- *Cook for 8 hours on low or 4 hours on high (slow cooker).*

Ingredients

- 2-pound beef chuck roast
- Salt and pepper to taste.
- Two teaspoons of vegetable oil.
- 1 onion, sliced
- 4 garlic cloves, minced
- Two tablespoons of soy sauce.
- 2 tablespoons Worcestershire sauce.
- 2 cups low-sodium beef broth.
- Four whole wheat hoagie rolls, split and toasted.
- Four slices of Provolone cheese

- Fresh parsley for garnish (optional).

Step-by-step instructions

- Salt and pepper the beef on both sides. Heat the oil in a big skillet over high heat. Sear the meat on all sides until browned, about 10 minutes. Transfer to a 6-quart slow cooker.

- Cook the onion and garlic in the same skillet over medium heat, turning periodically, until softened, about 10 minutes. Bring the soy sauce, Worcestershire sauce, and broth to a boil. Pour over the beef in the slow cooker.

- Cover and simmer on low for 8 hours or high for 4 hours, until the meat is soft and easily shredded with a fork.

- Place the beef on a cutting board and shred with two forks. Strain the cooking liquid and keep it for dipping.

- Divide the beef evenly between the bottom halves of the bread to make the sandwiches. Broil until the cheese is melted, which should take about 2 minutes.

- Sprinkle with parsley if desired. Serve alongside the reserved au jus for dipping. Enjoy!

Gyoza (Japanese Pot Stickers)

- _Servings: four._
- _Prepare time: 30 minutes._
- _Cook for 15 minutes._

Ingredients

- One-quarter pound ground pork
- Two cups finely chopped cabbage.
- Two green onions, minced
- One teaspoon of grated ginger.
- One teaspoon of soy sauce.
- A quarter teaspoon of sesame oil.
- Salt and pepper to taste.
- 24 gyoza wrappers.
- Two teaspoons of vegetable oil.
- One-quarter cup water
- Dipping sauce for serving.

Step-by-step instructions

- In a large mixing bowl, combine the pork, cabbage, green onions, ginger, soy sauce, sesame oil, salt, and pepper. Mix well with your hands until well blended.
- Place a gyoza wrapper on a lightly floured surface, then ladle about a spoonful of filling into the center. Moisten the

wrapper's edges with water before folding it in half and pleating the edges to seal. Repeat for the remaining wrappers and filling.

- Preheat the oil in a large skillet over medium-high heat. Cook the gyoza in a single layer in the skillet until the bottoms are brown, about 3 minutes.

- Add the water and cover with the lid. Steam for about 10 minutes, or until the water has evaporated and the gyoza are crispy.

- Transfer the gyoza to a plate and serve with your preferred dipping sauce. Enjoy!

Banh Mi (a Vietnamese sandwich)

- *Servings: four.*
- *Prep time is 20 minutes including marinating time.*
- *Cook for 10 minutes.*

Ingredients

- A quarter cup of rice vinegar
- Two teaspoons of sugar.
- One-quarter teaspoon of salt
- Two cups of shredded carrots.
- 2 cups shredded daikon radish.

- 1/4 cup mayonnaise.

- 2 teaspoons of Sriracha sauce.

- One pound of finely sliced pork tenderloin.

- Two tablespoons of soy sauce.

- Two tablespoons of fish sauce.

- Two teaspoons of lime juice.

- 2 garlic cloves, minced

- 1/4 teaspoon black pepper.

- Four whole wheat baguettes, sliced and toasted.

- A quarter cup of fresh cilantro leaves

- A quarter cup of fresh mint leaves

- 1/4 cup fresh basil leaves.

- 1 finely sliced jalapeño pepper (optional)

Step-by-step instructions

- In a small saucepan over medium heat, combine the vinegar, sugar, and salt. Whisk until the sugar dissolves. Bring to a boil, then remove from the heat and allow to cool slightly.

- In a large bowl, combine the carrots and daikon with the vinegar mixture. Refrigerate for at least 30 minutes, and up to overnight, stirring occasionally.

- In a small bowl, combine the mayonnaise and Sriracha sauce. Set aside.

- In a big Ziplock bag, mix together the pork, soy sauce, fish sauce, lime juice, garlic, and pepper. Seal the bag and massage to coat the meat.

- Refrigerate for at least 30 minutes, and up to overnight, turning the bag occasionally.

- Preheat a grill or grill pan to high heat. Remove the pork from the marinade and discard it. Grill the pork for about 2 minutes on each side, or until browned and well cooked. Transfer to a chopping board and let sit for 5 minutes. Slice thinly across the grain.

- To make the sandwiches, spread the mayonnaise mixture on the bottom halves of the baguettes. Top with pork, cilantro, mint, basil, and jalapeño (if using).

- Drain the carrot and daikon combination and place it on top of the herbs. Cover with the top half of the baguettes and enjoy!

Miso Ramen with Chashu Pork

- *Servings: four.*
- *Prep time is 15 minutes including marinating time.*
- *Cook for 45 minutes.*

Ingredients

- Cut 1 pound of pork belly into 1/4-inch-thick pieces.
- One-quarter cup soy sauce
- 1/4 cup mirin.
- Two teaspoons of brown sugar.
- Two teaspoons of miso paste.
- Four cups of chicken broth.
- Two teaspoons of miso paste.
- Two teaspoons of sesame oil.
- Four packages of instant ramen noodles.
- Four soft-boiled eggs, peeled and halved
- 4 green onions, sliced
- 4 sheets of nori seaweed cut into quarters.

Step-by-step instructions

- In a small bowl, combine the soy sauce, mirin, brown sugar, and miso paste. Put the pork pieces in a big Ziplock bag and pour in the marinade.
- Seal the bag and refrigerate for at least 2 hours or overnight, turning it occasionally.
- Preheat the oven to 375° Fahrenheit. Line a baking sheet with foil and coat with cooking spray. Place the pork slices in a single layer on the prepared baking sheet. Bake for 25

minutes, flipping halfway, until caramelized and well cooked.

- Heat the chicken stock in a large pot over medium-high heat until it boils. Whisk in the miso paste and sesame oil. Reduce the heat to a simmer for ten minutes.
- Cook the ramen noodles according to package directions, then drain and divide into four big bowls. Ladle the soup over the noodles, then top with the pork, eggs, green onions, and nori. Enjoy!

Garlic and Anchovy Pasta with Broccolini

- *Servings: four.*
- *Prep time is 10 minutes.*
- *Cook for 20 minutes.*

Ingredients

- 12 ounces of whole wheat spaghetti.
- Salt and pepper to taste.
- One-quarter cup olive oil
- 6 garlic cloves, thinly sliced
- Four anchovy fillets, chopped
- 1/4 teaspoon red pepper flakes.

- 1 bunch of broccolini (trimmed and sliced into bite-sized pieces)
- 1/4 cup grated parmesan cheese.
- 2 teaspoons of freshly chopped parsley.

Step-by-step instructions

- Heat a big saucepan of salted water to a boil. Cook the pasta until al dente, about 10 minutes. Reserve 1/2 cup of the cooking water and drain the pasta.
- Heat oil in a large skillet over medium-low heat. Cook, stirring, until the garlic is brown and the anchovies have dissolved, about 10 minutes.
- Simmer the broccolini with 1/4 cup of the saved pasta water. Cover and cook for approximately 5 minutes, or until the broccolini is crisp-tender.
- Add the pasta and stir to mix. If the sauce is too dry, add extra pasta water as needed. Season with salt and pepper to taste.
- Garnish with cheese and parsley and serve. Enjoy!

CHAPTER 5

<u>Poultry</u>

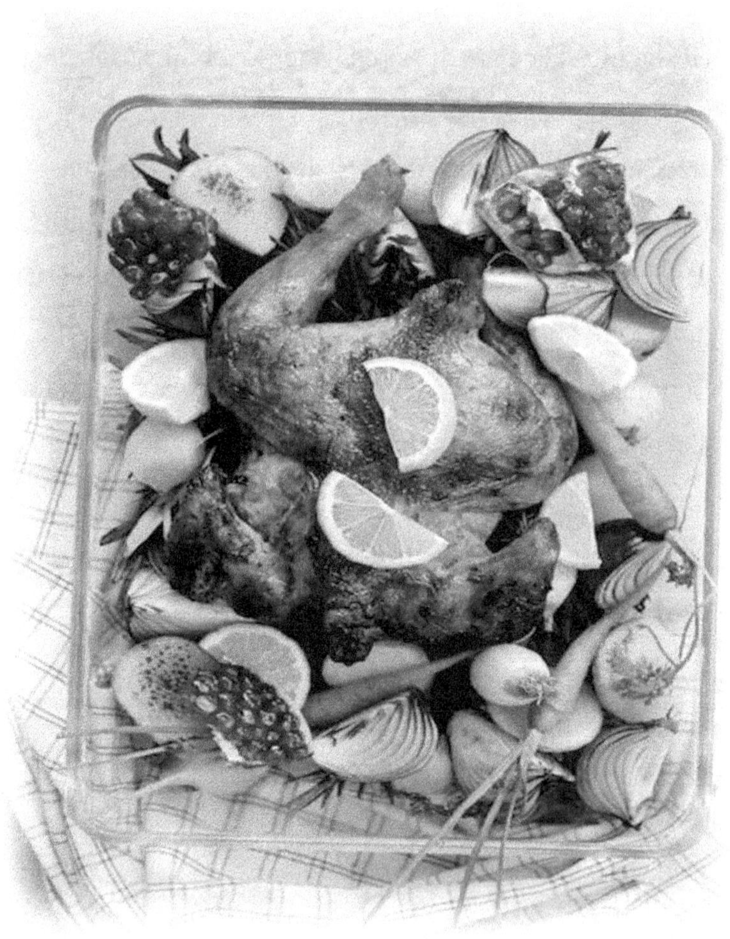

Chicken & Vegetable Soup

- *Servings: four.*
- *Prepare time: 15 minutes.*
- *Cook for 25 minutes.*

Ingredients:

- One tablespoon of olive oil.
- 1 onion, chopped
- 2 garlic cloves, minced
- Two carrots, peeled and chopped
- Two celery stalks, diced
- Four cups of chicken broth.
- Two bay leaves.
- One teaspoon dried thyme.
- Salt and pepper to taste.
- 2 chicken breasts, cooked and shredded
- Two cups of chopped spinach.
- 2 tablespoons chopped parsley.

Step-by-step Directions:

- Heat the oil in a big pot on medium-high heat. Cook the onion, garlic, carrots, and celery for about 10 minutes, stirring periodically, until tender.

- Boil the chicken broth, bay leaves, thyme, salt, and pepper. Reduce the heat to a simmer for about 15 minutes, or until the vegetables are soft.

- Cook for an additional 5 minutes, or until the spinach has wilted and the chicken is heated through.

- Remove the bay leaves and serve hot, or refrigerate in an airtight container for up to 3 days or freeze for up to 3 months.

Greek Chicken Salad with Lemon Dressing

- *Servings: four.*
- *Prep time is 20 minutes.*
- *Cook for 15 minutes.*

Ingredients:

For the Salad:

- 4 chicken breasts pounded to a consistent thickness.
- Salt and pepper to taste.
- Two teaspoons of dried oregano.
- Two teaspoons of olive oil.
- Eight cups of mixed greens.
- 1/4 cup sliced olives.
- 1/4 cup crumbled feta cheese.

- 1/4 cup chopped fresh dill.

For dressing:

- One-quarter cup olive oil
- One-quarter cup lemon juice
- Two teaspoons of honey.
- 1 teaspoon of Dijon mustard.
- One garlic clove, minced
- Salt and pepper to taste.

Step-by-step Directions:

- Sprinkle the chicken breasts with salt, pepper, and oregano on both sides. Heat the oil in a large skillet over medium-high heat.
- Cook the chicken for 7 minutes on each side, or until browned and cooked through. Transfer to a cutting board and rest for 5 minutes before slicing thinly.
- In a small bowl, mix together the dressing ingredients until thoroughly incorporated. Taste and adjust seasoning as needed.
- In a large salad bowl, combine the greens and half of the dressing. Divide the salad among four dishes, then top with the chicken, olives, feta, and dill.
- Drizzle the remaining dressing over the salads and serve, or refrigerate in separate airtight containers for up to two days.

Turkey Meatballs and Zucchini Noodles

- *Servings: four.*
- *Prepare time: 15 minutes.*
- *Cook for 20 minutes.*

Ingredients:

For meatballs:

- One pound of ground turkey.
- One-quarter cup almond flour
- One egg, lightly beaten
- 2 teaspoons of freshly chopped parsley.
- Two teaspoons of minced garlic.
- One teaspoon of salt.
- 1/2 teaspoon black pepper.
- 1/4 teaspoon red pepper flakes (optional).
- Two teaspoons of olive oil.

For zucchini noodles:

- Four medium zucchini spiralized or sliced into thin strips.
- Two teaspoons of olive oil.
- Salt and pepper to taste.
- 1/4 cup shredded parmesan cheese (optional)

Step-by-step Directions:

- In a large bowl, mix together the turkey, almond flour, egg, parsley, garlic, salt, pepper, and red pepper flakes (if using). Mix thoroughly and divide into 16 equal-sized meatballs.

- Preheat the oil in a large skillet over medium-high heat. Cook the meatballs for about 15 minutes, rotating regularly, until they are browned and cooked through. Transfer to a dish to keep heated.

- In the same skillet, heat the oil on medium-high heat. Cook the zucchini noodles, turning gently, for about 5 minutes, or until soft but still crisp. Season with salt and pepper to taste.

- Serve the zucchini noodles with the meatballs and parmesan cheese (if desired), or refrigerate in an airtight container for up to 3 days.

Roasted Chicken and Root Vegetables

- *Servings: four.*
- *Prepare time: 15 minutes.*
- *Cook for 45 minutes.*

Ingredients:

- One whole chicken (about 4 pounds), washed and patted dry
- Salt and pepper to taste.

- 2 tablespoons melted ghee or butter.

- Four fresh sprigs of rosemary

- 4 cloves of garlic, peeled and mashed

- Four medium potatoes, peeled and cut into bits

- Four medium carrots, peeled and cut into bits

- Two medium parsnips, peeled and sliced into bits

- Two teaspoons of olive oil.

- Two teaspoons dried thyme.

Step-by-step Directions:

- Preheat the oven to 375°F. Lightly butter a baking dish. Season the chicken cavity with salt and pepper, then stuff it with 2 sprigs of rosemary and 2 cloves garlic. Tie the legs together with kitchen twine, then tuck the wings under the torso.

- Brush the melted ghee or butter all over the chicken and season with additional salt and pepper.

- Place the chicken in the prepared baking dish and roast for 1 hour and 15 minutes, or until the skin is golden and crisp and the meat is fully cooked.

- A meat thermometer put into the thickest section of the thigh should register 165°F.

- In a large mixing basin, combine the potatoes, carrots, parsnips, olive oil, thyme, salt, and pepper. Place the vegetables in a single layer on a baking sheet and roast for about 45 minutes, or until soft and browned, flipping halfway through.

- Place the chicken on a chopping board and let it rest for 10 minutes before slicing. Serve over the roasted veggies and top with the remaining rosemary and garlic, or refrigerate in an airtight container for up to 3 days.

Chicken and Quinoa Stuffed Peppers

- *Servings: four.*
- *Prepare time: 15 minutes.*
- *Cook for 25 minutes.*

Ingredients:

- Four large bell peppers of any colour, halved and seeded.
- Two cups cooked quinoa.
- 2 cups shredded cooked chicken.
- 1/4 cup chopped fresh cilantro.
- One-quarter cup salsa
- Two teaspoons of cumin.
- One teaspoon of chili powder.
- Salt and pepper to taste.
- One cup shredded cheddar cheese.

- Sour cream to serve (optional)

Step-by-step Directions:

- Preheat the oven to 375°F. Lightly butter a baking dish. Place the pepper halves in the prepared dish, cut side up.

- In a large mixing bowl, add quinoa, chicken, cilantro, salsa, cumin, chili powder, salt, and pepper.

- Mix thoroughly and equally distribute the mixture among the pepper halves. Sprinkle the cheese over the top of the filling.

- Bake for approximately 25 minutes, or until the cheese has melted and the peppers are soft.

- Serve with sour cream (if desired), or refrigerate in an airtight container for up to three days.

Mediterranean Chicken with Rice Skillet

- *Servings: four.*
- *Prep time is 10 minutes.*
- *Cook for 25 minutes.*

Ingredients:

- Two teaspoons of olive oil.
- 4 chicken thighs, bone-in, skin-on
- Salt and pepper to taste.
- 1 onion, chopped

- 2 garlic cloves, minced
- One teaspoon of smoked paprika.
- 1/2 teaspoon dry oregano.
- 1/4 teaspoon red pepper flakes (optional).
- 1 1/2 cups chicken broth.
- 1 cup long-grain white rice.
- 1/4 cup chopped sun-dried tomatoes.
- 1/4 cup pitted Kalamata olives.
- 2 teaspoons of freshly chopped parsley.
- Two teaspoons of lemon juice.

Step-by-step Directions:

- Preheat the oil in a large skillet over medium-high heat. Season the chicken thighs with salt and pepper and place them on the skillet, skin side down. Cook for approximately 15 minutes, rotating once, or until golden and crisp. Transfer to a dish to keep heated.

- Reduce the heat to medium and stir in the onion, garlic, paprika, oregano, red pepper flakes (if using), and a pinch of salt and pepper. Cook for about 10 minutes, stirring periodically, until tender and aromatic.

- Bring the chicken stock and rice to a boil. Reduce the heat to a simmer, covered, for about 15 minutes, or until the rice is cooked and the liquid is absorbed.

- Combine sun-dried tomatoes, olives, parsley, and lemon juice. Place the chicken thighs on top of the rice and garnish with additional parsley if desired.
- Serve hot or refrigerate in an airtight container for up to three days.

Thai Chicken & Coconut Soup

- *Servings: four.*
- *Prepare time: 15 minutes.*
- *Cook for 20 minutes.*

Ingredients:

- One tablespoon of coconut oil.
- 1 onion, sliced
- 2 garlic cloves, minced
- One tablespoon of grated ginger.
- Two teaspoons of red or green curry paste.
- Four cups of chicken broth.
- One can of coconut milk (13.5 ounces)
- Two tablespoons of fish sauce.
- Two teaspoons of lime juice.
- Two teaspoons of honey or coconut sugar.
- Two finely cut chicken breasts.

- Two cups of sliced mushrooms.

- Two cups baby spinach.

- 1/4 cup chopped fresh cilantro.

- 1/4 cup chopped fresh basil.

Step-by-step Directions:

- Heat the oil in a big pot on medium-high heat. Cook the onion, garlic, ginger, and curry paste for about 10 minutes, stirring often, until the onion is tender and the curry paste is fragrant.

- Boil the chicken broth, coconut milk, fish sauce, lime juice, and coconut sugar or honey. Reduce the heat to a simmer for about 10 minutes, or until somewhat reduced.

- Add the chicken and mushrooms and heat for another 10 minutes, or until the chicken is fully cooked and the mushrooms are soft.

- Add the spinach, cilantro, and basil and simmer for another 5 minutes, or until wilted.

- Serve hot or refrigerate in an airtight container for up to three days.

Turkey Chili and Beans

- *Servings: six.*
- *Prep time is 10 minutes.*
- *Cook for 30 minutes.*

Ingredients:

- Two teaspoons of olive oil.
- One pound of ground turkey.
- Salt and pepper to taste.
- 1 onion, chopped
- 2 garlic cloves, minced
- Two tablespoons of chili powder.
- Two teaspoons of cumin.
- One teaspoon of oregano.
- 1/4 teaspoon cayenne pepper (optional).
- One (15-ounce) can of tomato sauce
- One can of chopped tomatoes (14.5 ounces)
- One can (15 ounces) of black beans, drained and rinsed
- 1 can (15 ounces) of drained and rinsed kidney beans.
- 1/4 cup chopped fresh cilantro.
- Serve with shredded cheese, sour cream, and green onions (optional).

Step-by-step Directions:

- Heat the oil in a big pot on medium-high heat. Cook the turkey, salt, and pepper for approximately 15 minutes, breaking it up with a wooden spoon, until browned and cooked through. Transfer to a dish to keep heated.

- In the same pot, combine the onion, garlic, chili powder, cumin, oregano, and cayenne pepper (if using) and simmer for 10 minutes, turning regularly, until the onion is tender and the spices are toasted.

- Boil the tomato sauce, diced tomatoes, black beans, kidney beans, and cilantro.

- Reduce the heat to a simmer, uncovered, for about 15 minutes, or until slightly thickened.

- Mix in the turkey and cook through. Serve with cheese, sour cream, and green onions (if desired), or chill in an airtight container in the refrigerator for up to 3 days or freeze for up to 3 months.

<u>*Chicken and Broccoli Stir-Fry*</u>

- *Servings: four.*
- *Prepare time: 15 minutes.*
- *Cook for 15 minutes.*

Ingredients:

For sauce:

- 1/4 cup low-sodium soy sauce.
- Two teaspoons of rice vinegar.
- Two teaspoons of honey.
- One spoonful of cornstarch.
- 1/4 teaspoon red pepper flakes (optional).

Prepare the stir-fry:

- Two teaspoons of sesame oil.
- Cut 1 pound of boneless, skinless chicken breasts into bite-sized pieces.
- Salt and pepper to taste.
- Four cups of broccoli florets.
- 2 garlic cloves, minced
- 2 tablespoons grated ginger.
- 2 tablespoons toasted sesame seeds.

Step-by-step Directions:

- In a small bowl, mix together the sauce ingredients until thoroughly incorporated. Set aside.

- Preheat the oil in a big skillet or wok over high heat. Season the chicken with salt and pepper, then add it to the skillet. Cook for about 10 minutes, stirring periodically, until golden and well cooked. Transfer to a dish to keep heated.

- In the same skillet, sauté the broccoli, garlic, ginger, and a splash of water for 5 minutes, turning often, until the broccoli is crisp-tender and the water has disappeared.

- Return the chicken to the skillet and pour in the sauce. Toss to coat and boil for an additional 5 minutes, or until the sauce thickens and bubbles.

- Sprinkle with sesame seeds and serve immediately, or refrigerate in an airtight container for up to three days.

CHAPTER 6

Soups And Stews.

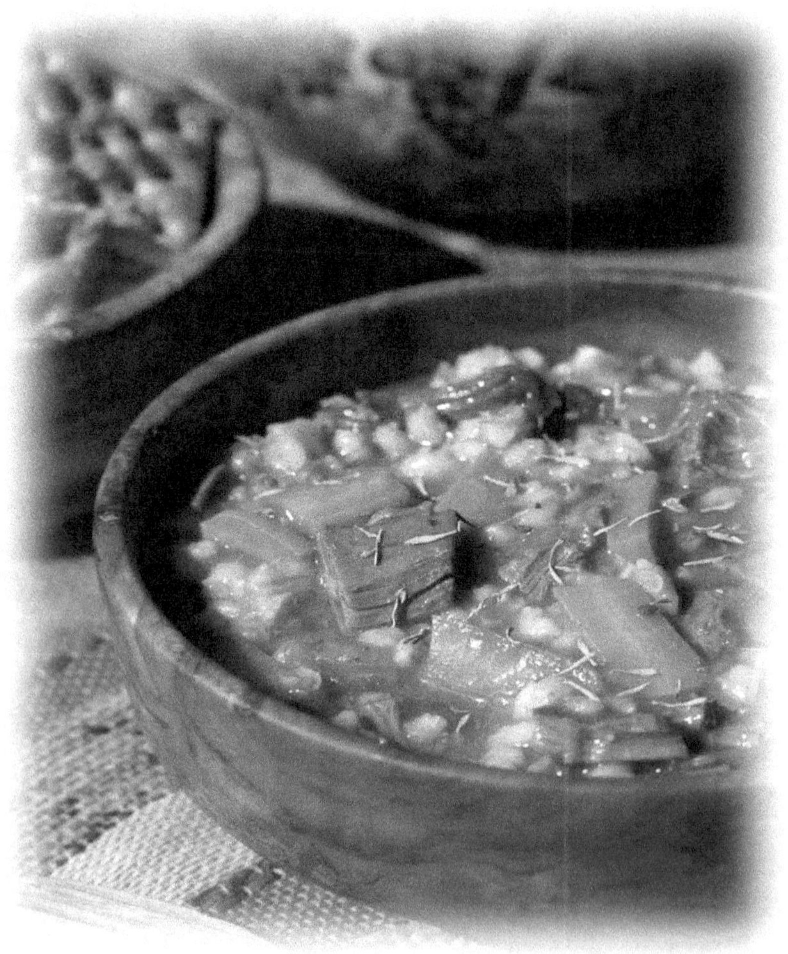

Roasted Tomato with Red Pepper Soup

- *Servings: four.*
- *Prep time is 10 minutes.*
- *Cook for 40 minutes.*

Ingredients:

- 2 pounds ripe tomatoes, halved.
- Two red bell peppers, seeded and quartered
- 4 garlic cloves, peeled
- Two teaspoons of olive oil.
- Salt and pepper to taste.
- Two cups of veggie broth.
- 1/4 cup fresh basil, chopped
- Two teaspoons of balsamic vinegar.

Instructions:

- Preheat the oven to 200 °C (400 °F) and line a baking sheet with parchment paper. Place the tomatoes, peppers, and garlic on the prepared baking sheet and sprinkle with olive oil. Season with salt and pepper to taste.
- Roast for 25–30 minutes, or until the tomatoes and peppers are tender and caramelized.
- Place the roasted veggies and any juices in a blender or food processor and mix until smooth.

- You may need to do this in batches, depending on the size of
  your blender or food processor.
- Transfer the pureed soup to a large pot and heat to a boil.
  Reduce the heat to a simmer for 10 minutes, stirring
  periodically.
- Stir in the basil and balsamic vinegar, and adjust the
  seasoning as needed.
- Serve hot, with crusty bread or croutons as preferred.

Mushroom and Leek Soup

- ***Servings: four.***
- ***Prepare time: 15 minutes.***
- ***Cook for 25 minutes.***

Ingredients:

- Two tablespoons of butter.
- Slice and rinse two leeks, only the white and light green
  sections.
- 2 garlic cloves, minced
- Four cups of sliced mushrooms (any variety)
- Two teaspoons of all-purpose flour.
- Four cups of veggie broth.
- One-quarter teaspoon dried thyme

- Salt and pepper to taste.

- A quarter cup of heavy cream or coconut milk

- 2 tablespoons fresh parsley, chopped

Instructions:

- Melt the butter in a large pot over medium-high heat. Cook for about 10 minutes, stirring occasionally, until the garlic and leeks are tender and wilted.

- Cook for an additional 10 minutes, until the mushrooms release their juices and brown slightly.

- Sprinkle the flour over the mushroom mixture and whisk to combine. Cook for 2 minutes, stirring regularly, to eliminate the raw flour taste.

- Gradually whisk in the vegetable broth, scraping away any brown pieces on the bottom of the pot. Add the thyme and season with salt and pepper to taste. Bring to a boil, then reduce heat and simmer for 15 minutes, until slightly thickened.

- Add the cream or coconut milk and parsley, and heat through, but do not boil.

- Serve hot, with more parsley if desired.

<u>*Lentil and Vegetable Soup*</u>

- *Servings: six.*
- *Prep time is 10 minutes.*
- *Cook for 40 minutes.*

Ingredients:

- Two teaspoons of olive oil.
- 1 onion, chopped
- Two carrots, peeled and chopped
- Two celery stalks, diced
- 2 garlic cloves, minced
- One teaspoon of cumin.
- 1/2 teaspoon turmeric.
- 1/4 teaspoon smoked paprika.
- Salt and pepper to taste.
- Rinse and drain 1 cup of brown or green lentils.
- Four cups of veggie broth.
- Two glasses of water.
- One bay leaf.
- 2 cups of chopped kale.
- Juice from 1 lemon

Instructions:

- Warm the olive oil in a big pot over medium-high heat. Cook the onion, carrots, celery, garlic, cumin, turmeric, smoked paprika, salt, and pepper for about 15 minutes, stirring occasionally, until the veggies are tender and fragrant.

- Bring the lentils, vegetable broth, water, and bay leaf to a boil. Reduce the heat to a simmer for 25 minutes, or until the lentils are cooked.

- Add the kale and lemon juice, and simmer for another 5 minutes, or until wilted.

- Remove the bay leaf and serve hot, with crusty bread or rice, as desired.

Roasted Butternut Squash Soup

- *Servings: four.*
- *Prepare time: 15 minutes.*
- *Cook for 45 minutes.*

Ingredients:

- One large butternut squash, peeled and cubed
- Two teaspoons of olive oil.
- Salt and pepper to taste.
- 1 onion, chopped

- 2 garlic cloves, minced

- Four cups of veggie broth.

- 1/4 teaspoon nutmeg.

- One-fourth teaspoon cinnamon

- A quarter cup of heavy cream or coconut milk

- Two teaspoons of maple syrup or honey.

- Fresh sage leaves as garnish (optional)

Instructions:

- Preheat the oven to 200 °C (400 °F) and line a baking sheet with parchment paper. Toss the squash cubes in 1 tablespoon olive oil and season with salt and pepper to taste. Spread them evenly on the prepared baking sheet and roast for 25 to 30 minutes, or until fork tender and caramelized.

- Heat the remaining olive oil in a large pot over medium-high heat. Sauté the onion and garlic for about 15 minutes, or until tender and translucent.

- Heat the vegetable broth, nutmeg, and cinnamon together until boiling. Reduce the heat to a simmer for 10 minutes, stirring periodically.

- Stir in the roasted squash and blend the soup with an immersion blender or in stages in a blender or food processor until smooth and creamy.

- Add the cream or coconut milk, maple syrup, or honey, and adjust the seasoning as needed.
- Serve hot and garnish with fresh sage leaves, if desired.

Curried Carrot and Chickpea Stew.

- **_Servings: four._**
- **_Prep time is 10 minutes._**
- **_Cook for 30 minutes._**

Ingredients:

- Two teaspoons of coconut oil.
- 1 onion, chopped
- 2 garlic cloves, minced
- 1 tablespoon of freshly grated ginger
- Two teaspoons of curry powder.
- One teaspoon of turmeric.
- 1/4 teaspoon cayenne pepper (optional).
- Salt and pepper to taste.
- Four cups of peeled and sliced carrots
- Two cups of veggie broth.
- One can of coconut milk, full-fat or light.
- One can of chickpeas, drained and rinsed
- Two cups baby spinach.

- 1/4 cup fresh cilantro, chopped
- Juice from 1 lime

Instructions:

- Melt the coconut oil in a large pot over medium-high heat. Cook the onion, garlic, ginger, curry powder, turmeric, cayenne pepper, salt, and pepper for about 10 minutes, stirring occasionally, until the onion is tender and fragrant.
- Bring the carrots and vegetable stock to a boil. Reduce the heat to a simmer for 15 minutes, or until the carrots are soft.
- Add the coconut milk and chickpeas, and bring to a boil again. Reduce the heat and simmer for a further 10 minutes, or until slightly thickened.
- Add the spinach, cilantro, and lime juice and simmer for another 5 minutes, or until wilted.
- Serve hot, with rice or naan bread, as preferred.

Cauliflower & Kale Soup

- *Servings: four.*
- *Prep time is 10 minutes.*
- *Cook for 25 minutes.*

Ingredients:

- Two teaspoons of olive oil.
- 1 onion, chopped
- 2 garlic cloves, minced
- Four cups of cauliflower florets.
- Four cups of veggie broth.
- One-quarter teaspoon dried thyme
- Salt and pepper to taste.
- 2 cups of chopped kale.
- 1/4 cup shredded Parmesan cheese (optional)

Instructions:

- Warm the olive oil in a big pot over medium-high heat. Cook the onion and garlic, stirring occasionally, for about 10 minutes, or until tender and transparent.
- Heat the cauliflower, vegetable broth, thyme, salt, and pepper till boiling. Reduce the heat to a simmer for 15 minutes, or until the cauliflower is fork-tender.

- Using an immersion blender or in batches in a blender or food processor, puree the soup until smooth and creamy.
- Add the kale and simmer for another 5 minutes, or until it is wilted.
- Serve hot, topped with Parmesan cheese if preferred.

Salmon & Sweet Potato Chowder

- ***Servings: four.***
- ***Prepare time: 15 minutes.***
- ***Cook for 25 minutes.***

Ingredients:

- Two tablespoons of butter.
- 1 onion, chopped
- Two celery stalks, diced
- 2 garlic cloves, minced
- Two teaspoons of all-purpose flour.
- Four cups of chicken broth.
- Two medium sweet potatoes, peeled and diced
- One-quarter teaspoon dried dill
- Salt and pepper to taste.
- 1 pound of skinless, boneless salmon fillets, cut into bite-sized pieces.

- A quarter cup of heavy cream or coconut milk

- 2 tablespoons fresh parsley, chopped

Instructions:

- Melt the butter in a large pot over medium-high heat. Stir in the onion, celery, and garlic and simmer for about 10 minutes, until the onion is tender and translucent.

- Sprinkle the flour over the onion mixture and mix thoroughly to coat. Cook for 2 minutes, stirring regularly, to eliminate the raw flour taste.

- Gradually whisk in the chicken broth, scraping away any brown pieces on the bottom of the pot. Bring the sweet potatoes, dill, salt, and pepper to a boil. Reduce the heat to a simmer for 15 minutes, or until the sweet potatoes are cooked.

- Cook for another 10 minutes, adding the salmon and cream or coconut milk, until the fish is fully cooked and the soup has thickened somewhat.

- Stir in the parsley and serve hot, with crusty bread or crackers as desired.

Lemony Chicken and Spinach Soup

- *Servings: four.*
- *Prep time is 10 minutes.*
- *Cook for 20 minutes.*

Ingredients:

- Two teaspoons of olive oil.
- 1 onion, chopped
- 2 garlic cloves, minced
- Four cups of chicken broth.
- Cut 2 chicken breasts into bite-size pieces.
- One-quarter teaspoon dried oregano
- Salt and pepper to taste.
- Two cups baby spinach.
- Juice and zest of one lemon
- 2 tablespoons fresh dill, chopped

Instructions:

- Warm the olive oil in a big pot over medium-high heat. Cook the onion and garlic, stirring occasionally, for about 10 minutes, or until tender and transparent.
- Boil the chicken broth, chicken, oregano, salt, and pepper. Reduce the heat to a simmer for 10 minutes, or until the chicken is cooked through.
- Add the spinach, lemon juice, lemon zest, and dill and simmer for another 5 minutes, or until wilted.
- Serve hot, with rice or couscous as preferred.

CHAPTER 7

<u>Vegetable Main Dishes</u>

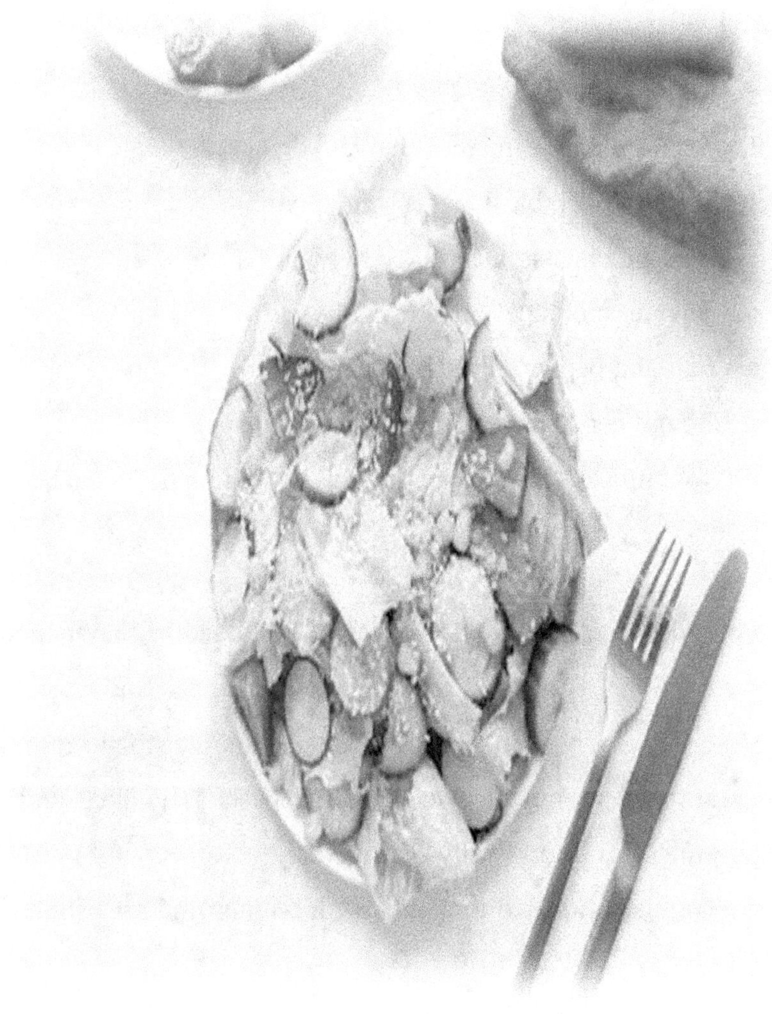

One-Pot Tomato Basil Pasta

- *Servings: four.*
- *Prepare time: 5 minutes.*
- *Cook for 20 minutes.*

Ingredients:

- 12 ounces of gluten-free or whole wheat spaghetti.
- 4 cups cherry tomatoes (halved)
- 1/4 cup fresh basil leaves, chopped
- 4 garlic cloves, thinly sliced
- Two teaspoons of olive oil.
- Salt and pepper to taste.
- Four cups of water.
- 1/4 cup shredded Parmesan cheese (optional)

Instructions:

- In a large pot over high heat, mix together the spaghetti, tomatoes, basil, garlic, olive oil, salt, pepper, and water.
- Bring to a boil, then reduce heat and simmer for 15 minutes, stirring periodically, or until the pasta is cooked and the water has been mostly absorbed.
- Garnish with Parmesan cheese if wanted and serve hot.

Pesto Ravioli with Spinach and Tomatoes.

- *Servings: four.*
- *Prep time is 10 minutes.*
- *Cook for 15 minutes.*

Ingredients:

- One container of cheese ravioli, fresh or frozen.
- Two cups baby spinach.
- One cup cherry tomato, halved
- 1/4 cup basil pesto.
- Salt and pepper to taste.

Instructions:

- Cook the ravioli per the package instructions, then drain and return to the saucepan.
- Toss together the spinach, tomatoes, pesto, salt, and pepper.
- Serve hot or cold, as preferred.

Easy Pea and Spinach Carbonara

- **Servings: four.**
- **Prep time is 10 minutes.**
- **Cook for 15 minutes.**

Ingredients:

- 12 ounces whole wheat or gluten-free penne
- Two cups frozen peas.
- 4 eggs
- A quarter cup of heavy cream or coconut milk
- 1/4 cup grated parmesan cheese.
- Salt and pepper to taste.
- Two cups baby spinach.

Instructions:

- Cook the penne according to package directions, then add the peas in the last 5 minutes. Drain and return to the pot.
- In a small bowl, combine the eggs, cream or coconut milk, Parmesan cheese, salt, and pepper.
- Toss the hot pasta and peas with the egg mixture until thoroughly coated. The heat from the pasta will cook the eggs, resulting in a creamy sauce.
- Stir in the spinach and serve hot, with additional Parmesan cheese if preferred.

Spinach and Avocado Smoothie

- *Servings: two.*
- *Prepare time: 5 minutes.*
- *Cook for 0 minutes.*

Ingredients:

- Two cups baby spinach.
- One ripe avocado, peeled and pitted
- One banana, peeled and sliced
- 2 cups almond milk (or water)
- Two tablespoons of honey or maple syrup.
- One-quarter teaspoon of vanilla extract
- Ice cubes (as needed)

Instructions:

- In a blender, mix the spinach, avocado, banana, almond milk or water, honey or maple syrup, and vanilla extract.
- Blend until smooth and creamy, adding ice cubes as needed to modify consistency and temperature.
- Pour into two glasses and enjoy!

White Bean and Sun-Dried Tomato Gnocchi

- *Servings: four.*
- *Prep time is 10 minutes.*
- *Cook for 15 minutes.*

Ingredients:

- One box of gnocchi (fresh or frozen).
- Two teaspoons of olive oil.
- 1/4 cup sun-dried tomatoes, chopped
- 2 garlic cloves, minced
- 1/4 teaspoon red pepper flakes (optional).
- Salt and pepper to taste.
- Two cups baby spinach.
- Drain and rinse one can of white beans.
- 1/4 cup shredded Parmesan cheese (optional)

Instructions:

- Cook the gnocchi according to package instructions, then drain and return it to the pot.
- Heat the olive oil in a large skillet over medium-high heat. Sauté the sun-dried tomatoes, garlic, red pepper flakes, salt, and pepper for 10 minutes, or until the tomatoes are soft and the garlic is fragrant.

- Cook for an additional 5 minutes, or until the spinach has wilted and the white beans are warm.
- Toss the gnocchi with the tomato-bean sauce, then top with Parmesan cheese, if preferred.
- Serve hot or cold, as preferred.

Spinach, Lima Beans, and Crispy Pancetta Pasta

- *Servings: four.*
- *Prep time is 10 minutes.*
- *Cook for 20 minutes.*

Ingredients:

- 12 ounces of gluten-free or whole wheat fusilli.
- 4 ounces of chopped pancetta.
- Two teaspoons of olive oil.
- 2 garlic cloves, minced
- Two cups of frozen lima beans.
- 4 cups baby spinach.
- Salt and pepper to taste.
- 1/4 cup shredded Parmesan cheese (optional)

Instructions:

- Cook the fusilli according to package instructions, then drain and return it to the pot.
- Cook the pancetta in a large skillet over medium-high heat, turning regularly, for 15 minutes, or until crisp and brown. Transfer to a plate lined with paper towels and let drain.
- In the same skillet, heat the olive oil and sauté the garlic for 5 minutes, or until tender and aromatic.
- Cook for an additional 10 minutes, until the lima beans are cooked and the spinach has wilted.
- Season with salt and pepper to taste.
- Toss the pasta with the bean-spinach mixture, then top with pancetta and Parmesan cheese, if preferred.
- Serve hot or cold, as preferred.

Garlic and Anchovy Pasta with Broccolini

- *Servings: four.*
- *Prep time is 10 minutes.*
- *Cook for 15 minutes.*

Ingredients:

- 12 ounces of gluten-free or whole wheat spaghetti.

- 1 bunch of broccolini (trimmed and sliced into bite-sized pieces)
- Two teaspoons of olive oil.
- Four anchovy fillets, chopped
- 4 garlic cloves, minced
- 1/4 teaspoon red pepper flakes (optional).
- Salt and pepper to taste.
- 2 tablespoons fresh parsley, chopped
- Two teaspoons of lemon juice.

Instructions:

- Cook the pasta according to package directions, then add the broccolini in the last 5 minutes. Drain and return to the pot.
- In a small skillet over medium-low heat, heat the olive oil and sauté the anchovies, garlic, red pepper flakes, salt, and pepper for 10 minutes, stirring periodically, until the anchovies dissolve and the garlic turns golden.
- Toss the anchovy-garlic mixture with the spaghetti and broccolini until well combined.
- Garnish with parsley and lemon juice and serve hot.

Creamy White Chili with Cream Cheese

- *Servings: six.*
- *Prep time is 10 minutes.*
- *Cook for 30 minutes.*

Ingredients:

- Two tablespoons of butter.
- 1 onion, chopped
- 2 garlic cloves, minced
- Four cups of veggie broth.
- Drain and rinse two cans of white beans.
- 1 can of chopped green chiles.
- One teaspoon of cumin.
- 1/2 teaspoon oregano.
- Salt and pepper to taste.
- 8 ounces cream cheese, cubed
- 1/4 cup fresh cilantro, chopped

Instructions:

- Melt the butter in a large pot over medium-high heat. Cook the onion and garlic, stirring occasionally, for about 10 minutes, or until tender and transparent.
- Boil the vegetable broth, white beans, green chilies, cumin, oregano, salt, and pepper.

- Reduce the heat to a simmer for 15 minutes, stirring occasionally.
- Add the cream cheese and heat for a further 5 minutes, or until melted and smooth.
- Add the cilantro and serve hot with your preferred toppings, such as cheese, sour cream, avocado, or tortilla chips.

Seared Scallops with Green Goddess Slaw.

- *Servings: four.*
- *Prepare time: 15 minutes.*
- *Cook for 10 minutes.*

Ingredients:

- One-quarter cup plain yogurt
- Two tablespoons of mayonnaise.
- 2 tablespoons fresh parsley, chopped
- 2 tablespoons fresh tarragon, chopped
- 2 teaspoons of freshly chopped chives.
- Two teaspoons of lemon juice.
- Salt and pepper to taste.
- Four cups of shredded cabbage.
- Two carrots, peeled and shredded
- 1/4 cup sliced almonds, toasted

- Two teaspoons of olive oil.
- 1 pound of scallops, pat dry.

Instructions:

- In a small mixing bowl, combine the yogurt, mayonnaise, parsley, tarragon, chives, lemon juice, salt, and pepper. This is the green goddess dressing.
- In a large bowl, combine the cabbage, carrots, and almonds with half of the dressing. This is the coleslaw.
- Heat the olive oil in a large skillet over high heat, then sear the scallops for about 3 minutes on each side, until golden and cooked through. Season with salt and pepper to taste.
- Arrange the scallops on top of the slaw and sprinkle with the remaining dressing.

Orange-Mint Freekeh Salad with Lima beans

- *Servings: four.*
- *Prep time is 10 minutes.*
- *Cook for 20 minutes.*

Ingredients:

- 1 cup freekeh, rinsed and drained.

- Two cups of veggie broth.

- Two oranges, peeled and segmented

- 1/4 cup fresh mint leaves, chopped

- Two teaspoons of olive oil.

- Two teaspoons of apple cider vinegar.

- Salt and pepper to taste.

- Two cups of frozen lima beans.

- 4 cups baby spinach.

Instructions:

- Heat a medium pot over high heat and bring the freekeh and vegetable broth to a boil.

- Reduce the heat to a simmer for 20 minutes, or until the freekeh is soft and the liquid is absorbed. Fluff with a fork before transferring to a large bowl.

- Toss the oranges, mint, olive oil, vinegar, salt, and pepper until well combined.

- In a small pot over medium-high heat, boil the lima beans for 10 minutes, or until cooked. Drain and mix into the freekeh salad.

- Serve the salad hot or cold over a bed of spinach.

CHAPTER 8

Seafood

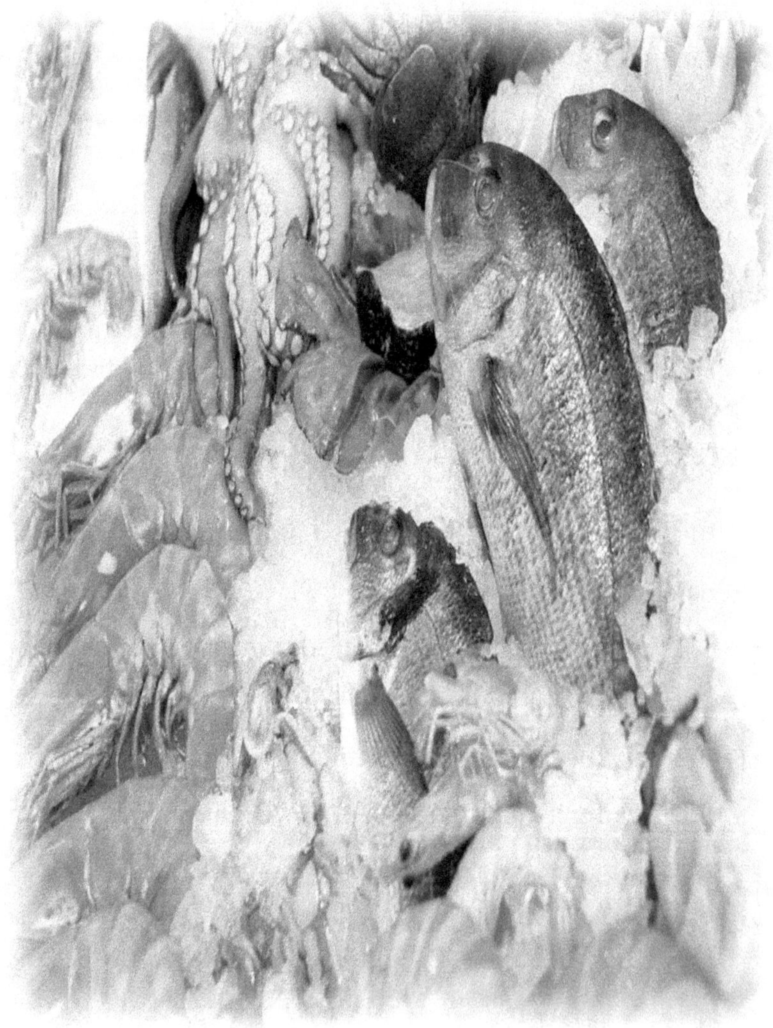

Omega-3-Rich Baked Salmon

- *Servings: four.*
- *Prep time is 10 minutes.*
- *Cook for 15 minutes.*

Ingredients:

- Four salmon fillets, skinless and boneless
- Salt and pepper to taste.
- 2 tablespoons Dijon mustard.
- Two teaspoons of honey.
- Two teaspoons of lemon juice.
- 2 garlic cloves, minced
- 2 tablespoons fresh rosemary, chopped
- Two teaspoons of olive oil.
- 4 cups baby spinach.

Instructions:

- Preheat the oven to 200 °C (400 °F) and line a baking sheet with parchment paper. Season the salmon fillets with salt and pepper, then arrange them on the prepared baking sheet.
- In a small bowl, combine the mustard, honey, lemon juice, garlic, and rosemary. Spoon the mixture over the salmon fillets, distributing evenly.

- Bake for 15 minutes, or until salmon is flaky and fully cooked.

- In a large skillet over medium-high heat, heat the olive oil and sauté the spinach for 5 minutes, or until wilted. Season with salt and pepper to taste.

- Place the salmon over a bed of spinach and sprinkle with any leftover sauce from the baking sheet.

Shrimp and Avocado Salad

- *Servings: four.*
- *Prepare time: 15 minutes.*
- *Cook for 10 minutes.*

Ingredients:

- One pound of peeled and deveined shrimp.
- Salt and pepper to taste.
- Two teaspoons of olive oil.
- •Two avocados, peeled and diced
- 2 cups cherry tomatoes, halved
- 1/4 cup fresh cilantro, chopped
- Two teaspoons of lime juice.
- One-quarter teaspoon of cumin
- One-quarter teaspoon of chili powder

Instructions:

- Season the shrimp with salt and pepper. Heat the olive oil in a large skillet over high heat, then cook the shrimp for 5 minutes, flipping once, until pink and cooked through. Transfer to a large bowl and allow it cool somewhat.
- Toss the avocados, tomatoes, cilantro, lime juice, cumin, and chili powder into the bowl with the shrimp until well combined.
- Serve chilled or at room temperature, as a salad or wrap filling.

Grilled Salmon Fillet

- ***Servings: four.***
- ***Prep time is 10 minutes.***
- ***Cook for 10 minutes.***

Ingredients:

- Four salmon fillets, skinless and boneless
- Two tablespoons of soy sauce.
- Two teaspoons of honey.
- One tablespoon of sesame oil.
- 1 tablespoon of freshly grated ginger
- 2 garlic cloves, minced

- 1/4 teaspoon black pepper.
- 2 teaspoons of toasted sesame seeds.
- 2 green onions, sliced

Instructions:

- In a small mixing bowl, combine the soy sauce, honey, sesame oil, ginger, garlic, and pepper. This is the marinade.
- Put the salmon fillets in a shallow dish and pour the marinade over them. Turn to coat thoroughly and chill for at least 30 minutes, or up to 2 hours.
- Preheat a grill or grill pan over medium-high heat, then generously oil the grate.
- Remove the salmon from the marinade, shaking off any excess. Save the marinade for later.
- Grill the salmon for about 5 minutes on each side, or until it flakes easily with a fork. Brush on the saved marinade halfway through cooking.
- Garnish with sesame seeds and green onions and serve hot.

Tequila Lime Shrimp Zoodles.

- *Servings: four.*
- *Prepare time: 15 minutes.*
- *Cook for 15 minutes.*

Ingredients:

- 4 medium zucchinis spiralized or sliced into thin noodles.
- Salt and pepper to taste.
- Two teaspoons of olive oil.
- One pound of peeled and deveined shrimp.
- Two tablespoons of tequila.
- Two teaspoons of lime juice.
- 2 garlic cloves, minced
- 1/4 teaspoon red pepper flakes (optional).
- 2 tablespoons fresh cilantro, chopped

Instructions:

- Place the zucchini noodles in a colander and season with salt. Allow them to drain for 10 minutes before squeezing out any extra water with paper towels.
- Heat the olive oil in a big skillet over high heat, then cook the shrimp for about 5 minutes, flipping once, until pink and fully done. Transfer to a dish to keep heated.

- In the same skillet, combine the tequila, lime juice, garlic, red pepper flakes, salt, and pepper and heat until boiling.
- Reduce the heat to a simmer for 5 minutes, stirring regularly, until somewhat reduced.
- Stir in the zucchini noodles and cilantro until fully combined. Cook for an additional 5 minutes, or until the noodles are well heated and coated in sauce.
- Top the zoodles with the shrimp and more cilantro, if desired.

Lemony Scallops and Angel Hair Pasta

- *Servings: four.*
- *Prep time is 10 minutes.*
- *Cook for 15 minutes.*

Ingredients:

- 12 ounces of whole wheat or gluten-free angel hair pasta.
- Two tablespoons of butter.
- 1 pound of scallops, pat dry.
- Salt and pepper to taste.
- Two teaspoons of olive oil.
- 2 garlic cloves, minced
- A quarter cup of white wine or chicken broth

- Two teaspoons of lemon juice.
- 2 tablespoons fresh parsley, chopped
- 2 teaspoons of drained capers.

Instructions:

- Cook the pasta according to package instructions, then drain and return it to the saucepan.
- Melt the butter in a large skillet over high heat, then sear the scallops for about 3 minutes on each side, until golden and cooked through. Season with salt and pepper to taste. Transfer to a dish to keep heated.
- In the same skillet, heat the olive oil and sauté the garlic for 5 minutes, or until tender and aromatic.
- Heat the wine or broth, lemon juice, parsley, and capers until boiling. Reduce the heat to a simmer for 5 minutes, stirring occasionally, until slightly thickened.
- Serve the pasta topped with the scallops and sauce.

Air fryer Fish and Chips

- *Servings: four.*
- *Prepare time: 15 minutes.*
- *Cook for 15 minutes.*

Ingredients:

- Four medium potatoes, peeled and sliced into thin wedges
- Two teaspoons of olive oil.
- Salt and pepper to taste.
- One-quarter cup cornstarch
- One-quarter cup water
- One-quarter teaspoon of baking powder
- 1/4 teaspoon paprika.
- One-quarter teaspoon of garlic powder
- One-quarter teaspoon of onion powder
- Four cod fillets, skinless and boneless

Cooking Spray

- Tartar sauce to serve (optional).
- Lemon wedges to serve (optional)

Instructions:

- Preheat an air fryer to 200°C (400°F), then spray the basket with cooking spray.
- In a large dish, toss the potato wedges with olive oil and season with salt and pepper to taste.
- Place them in a single layer in the air fryer basket and cook for 15 minutes, flipping halfway through, until golden and crispy.
- In a small mixing bowl, combine the cornstarch, water, baking powder, paprika, garlic powder, onion powder, salt, and pepper. This is the batter.
- Dip the cod fillets into the batter, shaking off any excess. Put them on a plate and spray both sides with cooking spray.
- Take the potato wedges out of the air fryer and keep warm. Place the cod fillets in the same basket and cook for 10 minutes, flipping halfway, or until brown and flaky.
- Optional: Serve the fish and chips with tartar sauce and lemon wedges.

Halibut Soft Tacos

- *Servings: four.*
- *Prep time is 10 minutes.*
- *Cook for 10 minutes.*

Ingredients:

- One-quarter cup plain yogurt
- Two tablespoons of mayonnaise.
- Two teaspoons of lime juice.
- One-quarter teaspoon of cumin
- Salt and pepper to taste.
- 1/4 cup fresh cilantro, chopped
- 1/4 cup fresh mint, chopped
- 1 pound of halibut fillets, skinless and boneless
- Two teaspoons of olive oil.
- Eight warmed corn or wheat tortillas.
- Two cups of shredded cabbage.
- 1/4 cup sliced radishes.

Instructions:

- In a small bowl, combine the yogurt, mayonnaise, lime juice, cumin, salt, and pepper. This is a yogurt sauce.
- In another small bowl, combine the cilantro and mint. This is the herbal concoction.

- Season halibut fillets with salt and pepper. In a large skillet over medium-high heat, heat the olive oil and fry the halibut for 5 minutes per side, or until brown and cooked through. Flake with a fork and place on a dish.

- To build the tacos, spread some yogurt sauce on each tortilla, then top with halibut, cabbage, radishes, and herb mixture. Fold, and enjoy!

Seafood Stir Fry

- *Servings: four.*
- *Prepare time: 15 minutes.*
- *Cook for 15 minutes.*

Ingredients:

- Two tablespoons of soy sauce.
- One spoonful of honey.
- One spoonful of cornstarch.
- One-quarter teaspoon ginger
- One-quarter teaspoon of garlic powder
- 1/4 teaspoon red pepper flakes (optional).
- Cut 1 pound of mixed seafood, such as shrimp, scallops, squid, or fish, into bite-sized pieces.
- Two teaspoons of vegetable oil.

- 4 cups chopped mixed veggies, including broccoli, carrots, snow peas, or bell peppers.
- Two cups cooked brown rice or quinoa.

Instructions:

- In a small mixing bowl, combine the soy sauce, honey, cornstarch, ginger, garlic powder, and red pepper flakes. This is the sauce.
- Heat the oil in a big skillet over high heat, then stir-fry the seafood for 10 minutes, or until cooked through and golden. Transfer to a dish to keep heated.
- In the same skillet, cook the vegetables for about 10 minutes, or until crisp-tender.
- Toss the seafood and sauce together until fully coated. Cook for a further 5 minutes, or until the sauce thickens and bubbles.
- Serve the stir-fry with rice or quinoa, if desired.

Shrimp and Broccoli Spaghetti Squash Alfredo

- *Servings: four.*
- *Prepare time: 15 minutes.*
- *Cook for 45 minutes.*

Ingredients:

- 1 large spaghetti squash halved and seeded.
- Two teaspoons of olive oil.
- Salt and pepper to taste.
- One-quarter cup butter
- 2 garlic cloves, minced
- 1/4 cup all-purpose flour.
- Two glasses of milk.
- 1/4 teaspoon nutmeg.
- 1/4 cup grated parmesan cheese.
- One pound of peeled and deveined shrimp.
- 2 cups steamed broccoli florets.
- 2 tablespoons fresh parsley, chopped

Instructions:

- Preheat the oven to 200 °C (400 °F) and line a baking sheet with parchment paper. Drizzle olive oil over the spaghetti squash halves and season with salt and pepper to taste. Place them cut side down on the prepared baking sheet and bake for 40 minutes, or until soft.

- In a medium saucepan over medium-low heat, melt the butter and sauté the garlic for 5 minutes, or until tender and aromatic.
- Whisk in the flour and simmer for 2 minutes, stirring constantly, to eliminate the raw flour taste.
- Bring the milk, nutmeg, salt, and pepper to a boil while whisking in gradually. Reduce the heat to a simmer for 10 minutes, stirring periodically, until slightly thickened.
- Add the Parmesan cheese and keep heated. This is the Alfredo sauce.
- Cook the shrimp in a large skillet over high heat for 5 minutes, stirring once, until pink and cooked through. Season with salt and pepper to taste.
- Using a fork, scrape the spaghetti squash strands into a big bowl. Toss in the Alfredo sauce, shrimp, and broccoli until completely combined.
- Garnish with parsley and serve hot.

Tomato Basil Cod with Asparagus.

- *Servings: four.*
- *Prep time is 10 minutes.*
- *Cook for 20 minutes.*

Ingredients:

- Four cod fillets, skinless and boneless
- Salt and pepper to taste.
- Two teaspoons of olive oil.
- 4 garlic cloves, minced
- A quarter cup of white wine or chicken broth
- 2 cups cherry tomatoes, halved
- 1/4 cup fresh basil leaves, chopped
- 1 pound asparagus, trimmed and divided into thirds
- Two tablespoons of butter.
- Two teaspoons of lemon juice.

Instructions:

- Season the cod filets with salt and pepper. In a large skillet over medium-high heat, heat the olive oil and fry the cod for 10 minutes, flipping once, until brown and flaky. Transfer to a dish to keep heated.

- In the same skillet, combine the garlic and wine or broth and heat to a boil. Reduce the heat to a simmer for 5 minutes, scraping up any brown bits from the bottom of the pan.
- Cook for an additional 5 minutes, until the tomatoes are mushy and the sauce has thickened slightly.
- Cook the asparagus in a small pot of boiling water for about 5 minutes, or until it is crisp tender. Drain and return to the pot.
- Toss in the butter and lemon juice until evenly coated. Season with salt and pepper to taste.
- Serve the fish topped with the tomato-basil sauce and asparagus.

CHAPTER 9

2-Week Meal Plan

Week 1

Day 1

- Breakfast: Kefir, banana, almond, and frozen berry smoothie.
- Snack: handful of almonds and dried apricots.
- Lunch is Greek chicken salad with lemon dressing.
- Snack: carrot sticks with hummus.
- Dinner: Cassoulet Recipe

Day 2

- Breakfast: Spring greens shakshuka.
- Snack: Hard-boiled egg and apple.
- Lunch: Turkey chili and beans.
- Snack: celery sticks with peanut butter.
- Dinner is grilled salmon fillet.

Day 3

- Breakfast: vegan overnight oats.
- Snack: Banana and granola bar.

- Lunch: roasted tomato and red pepper soup.

- Snack: Yogurt with berries

- Dinner is bratwurst and sauerkraut.

Day 4

- Breakfast: figs on toast with goat yogurt labneh.

- Snack: handful of walnuts and raisins.

- Lunch is mushroom and leek soup.

- Snack: cheese and crackers.

- Dinner: Tequila Lime Shrimp Zoodles

Day 5

- Breakfast: Miso chickpeas with avocado on toast.

- Snack: Pear and string cheese.

- Lunch is lentil and vegetable soup.

- Snack: popcorn with dark chocolate.

- Dinner: Air fryer (pork schnitzel with mushroom gravy).

Day 6

- Breakfast: Healthy banana pancakes.

- Snacks: kiwi and muffin.

- Lunch is roasted butternut squash soup.

- Snack: Edamame with dried cranberries.

- Dinner: french dip sandwich.

Day 7

- Breakfast: Raspberry, peach, and mango smoothie bowl.
- Snack: One slice of banana bread and a glass of milk.
- Lunch: curried carrot and chickpea stew.
- Snack: Peach and pistachios.
- Dinner: Gyoza (Japanese potstickers).

Week 2

Day 8

- Breakfast is white bean and avocado toast.
- Snack: One grapefruit and a handful of cashews
- Lunch: Cauliflower and Kale Soup
- Snack: carrot cake with a cup of tea.
- Dinner: Banh mi (a Vietnamese sandwich).

Day 9

- Breakfast: berry-kefir smoothie.
- Snack: Hard-boiled egg and orange.
- Lunch: Salmon with sweet potato chowder
- Snack: cucumber slices with tzatziki.
- Dinner: Miso ramen with chashu pork

Day 10

- Breakfast: chocolate banana oatmeal.
- Snack: Blueberry muffin and glass of milk.
- Lunch is lemony chicken and spinach soup.
- Snack: One handful of trail mix.
- Dinner: Garlic and anchovy spaghetti with broccolini

Day 11

- Breakfast: Kefir, banana, almond, and frozen berry smoothie.
- Snack: handful of almonds and dried apricots.
- Lunch is chicken and vegetable soup.
- Snack: carrot sticks with hummus.
- Dinner: White bean and sun-dried tomato gnocchi.

Day 12

- Breakfast: Spring greens shakshuka.
- Snack: Hard-boiled egg and apple.
- Lunch is Greek chicken salad with lemon dressing.
- Snack: celery sticks with peanut butter.
- Dinner: Spinach, lima beans, and crispy pancetta pasta.

Day 13

- Breakfast: vegan overnight oats.

- Snack: Banana and granola bar.
- Lunch: Turkey meatballs and zucchini noodles.
- Snack: Yogurt with berries
- Dinner: Lemony scallops and angel hair pasta.

Day 14

- Breakfast: figs on toast with goat yogurt labneh.
- Snack: handful of walnuts and raisins.
- Lunch: Roasted chicken and root veggies.
- Snack: cheese and crackers.
- Dinner: air-fried fish and chips.

Shopping List for Gut Health Diet

Top Gut-Friendly Ingredients

These are some of the foods that are very helpful for your gut health because they include nutrients or substances that feed your friendly bacteria, stimulate digestion, or reduce inflammation.

Prebiotics

Prebiotics are fibres that act as food for gut bacteria, allowing them to grow and thrive. Some of the most effective sources of prebiotics are:

- Onions

- Garlic.

- Leeks.

- The asparagus

- Artichokes.

- Bananas

- Oats

- Barley

- Flaxseeds.

- Apples.

- Chicory root.

- Dandelion greens.

Probiotics

Probiotics are meals or pills that contain live cultures of helpful bacteria. They can help restore your gut flora and improve your digestion. Some of the most effective sources of probiotics are:

- Yogurt

- Kefir.

- Sauerkraut.

- Kimchi.

- Miso

- Tempeh.

- Kombucha.

- Pickles
- Natto.
- Sourdough bread.

Fiber

Fiber is a carbohydrate that your body cannot digest, but intestinal microorganisms can. Fiber helps to regulate bowel movements, decrease cholesterol, and control blood sugar.

Fiber also makes you feel full and content, which can help you avoid binge eating and weight gain. Some of the best sources of fiber include:

- Fruits
- Vegetables
- Whole grains.
- Legumes.
- Nuts
- Seeds

Antioxidants

Antioxidants are compounds that protect your cells from free radical damage, which is caused by unstable molecules that can lead to inflammation and disease. Antioxidants also boost your immune system and help you avoid illnesses. Here are some of the best antioxidant sources:

- Berries
- Citrus Fruits
- Grapes
- Pomegranates.
- Tomatoes
- Carrots.
- Spinach.
- Kale
- Broccoli
- Brussels Sprouts
- Cauliflower
- Cabbage.
- Turmeric
- Ginger.
- Green tea.
- Dark chocolate.
- Red wine.

Anti-inflammatory

Anti-inflammatory foods are those that can help reduce inflammation in the body, which has been associated to a variety of chronic illnesses, including diabetes, obesity, heart disease, and cancer.

Anti-inflammatory foods can also help to soothe your gut and prevent or alleviate symptoms of IBS, IBD, and gastritis. Some of the most effective anti-inflammatory meals are:

- Fatty fish.
- Olive Oil.
- Avocado.
- Nuts
- Seeds
- Garlic.
- Onion
- Turmeric
- Ginger.
- Cinnamon.
- Rosemary.
- Thyme.
- Oregano.
- Basil.
- Mint
- Parsley.
- Coriander

Stocking A Gut-Friendly Pantry

These are some of the foods that can be stored in your pantry or freezer for ease and diversity. They can assist you in preparing healthy and convenient meals or snacks.

Complex carbohydrates

Complex carbs have a complex structure and take longer to digest, giving you long-lasting energy and keeping your blood sugar constant.

Complex carbohydrates contain more fiber, vitamins, minerals, and phytochemicals than simple carbs, which have been refined and processed. Here are some of the top sources of complex carbohydrates:

- Gluten-free or whole wheat pasta.
- Brown Rice
- Quinoa
- Buckwheat.
- Millet.
- Oats
- Barley
- Spelled
- Rye
- Amaranth.

- Teff

- Sorghum.

- Corn

- Potatoes

- Sweet Potatoes

- Squash.

- A pumpkin.

Protein

Protein is a macronutrient that your body requires to produce and repair its tissues, muscles, organs, and enzymes. Protein also makes you feel full and satisfied, preventing overeating and weight gain.

Protein also helps your immune system fend off infections. Here are some of the top sources of protein:

- Eggs
- Chicken
- Turkey.
- Beef
- Pork
- Lamb
- Fish
- Shellfish.
- Tofu
- Tempeh.

- Edamame.

- Beans

- Lentils.

- Chickpeas.

- Peas

- Peanut Butter.

- Almond Butter

- Cashew Butter

- Sunflower Seed Butter

- Tahini.

- Cheese

- Cottage Cheese.

- Ricotta Cheese

- Mozzarella Cheese

- Feta Cheese

- Goat Cheese

- Parmesan cheese.

- Cheddar Cheese

- Swiss Cheese

Healthy fats.

Healthy fats are those that are unsaturated or include omega-3 fatty acids, which can help lower cholesterol, improve heart health, and decrease inflammation.

Healthy fats also help you absorb fat-soluble vitamins including A, D, E, and K. Healthy fats also keep you energized and satiated. Some of the top sources of healthy fats are:

- Olive Oil.
- Coconut Oil
- Avocado oil.
- Sesame oil.
- Flaxseed oil.
- Walnut Oil
- Canola oil.
- Sunflower oil.
- Safflower oil.
- Peanut oil.
- Avocado.
- Olives.
- Nuts
- Seeds
- Flaxseeds.
- Chia Seeds

- Hemp Seeds

- Pumpkin Seeds

- Sunflower Seeds

- Sesame Seeds

- Walnuts.

- Almonds.

- Cashews.

- Pistachios.

- Pecans.

- Macadamia nuts.

- Brazilian nuts

- Pine nuts.

Pantry staples and frozen foods

These are some of the foods that can be stored in your pantry or freezer for ease and diversity. They can assist you in preparing healthy and convenient meals or snacks.

- Canned or jarred tomatoes.

- Tomato paste.

- Tomato Sauce

- Salsa.

- Marinara sauce.

- Pesto Sauce

- Alfredo Sauce

- Soy Sauce.

- Tamari sauce.

- Teriyaki Sauce

- Hoisin sauce.

- Oyster Sauce

- Fish Sauce

- Worcestershire Sauce

- Barbeque sauce

- Ketchup.

- Mustard.

- Mayonnaise.

- Salad dressing.

- Vinegar

- Balsamic vinegar.

- Apple Cider Vinegar

- Rice Vinegar

- White wine vinegar.

- Red wine vinegar.

- Champagne vinegar

- Honey.

- Maple syrup.

- Molasses.

- Agave nectar.

- Sugar.

- Brown sugar.

- Powdered sugar.

- Coconut sugar.

- Stevia

- Salt

- Black pepper.

- Red pepper flakes.

- Paprika.

- Smoked paprika.

- Cayenne Pepper

- Chili Powder

- Curry Powder.

- Turmeric

- Cumin

- Coriander

- Cardamom.

- Cinnamon.

- Nutmeg.

- Clove.

- Parsley.

- Coriander

- Baking Powder

- Cornstarch.

- Flour

- Whole wheat flour.

- All-purpose flour.

- Bread flour.

- Cake flour.

- Quinoa Flour

- Teff Flour

- Sorghum Flour

- Corn meal.

- Polenta.

- Grits.

- Couscous.

- Bulgur.

- Frozen Fruit

- Frozen veggies.

- Frozen meat.

- Frozen seafood.

- Frozen pizza.

Your gut encompasses more than just your stomach. It is a complicated network of organs and bacteria that influences your digestion, immunity, mood, and overall health.

To keep your gut healthy and happy, eat a well-balanced diet, supplement with probiotics, and exercise often.

Exercise can improve your gut health in a variety of ways, including:

- Improving gut motility, or the flow of food and waste through the digestive tract. This can help avoid constipation, bloating, and other digestive disorders.
- Increased blood circulation, which brings more oxygen and nutrients to your intestines and other organs. This can improve the operation and health of your intestinal cells and bacteria.
- Toning your abdominal muscles can help support your digestive organs and reduce belly fat. Belly obesity can promote inflammation and disturb the balance of bacteria in your gut, known as the microbiome.
- Reducing stress, which can have a detrimental impact on gut health and induce symptoms like diarrhea, nausea, or loss of

appetite. Exercise helps reduce cortisol levels, a stress hormone that can hurt your gut.

To gain the benefits of exercise for your gut, aim for at least 150 minutes of moderate-intensity aerobic activity per week, such as walking, running, cycling, or swimming. To improve your muscular tone and posture, incorporate some strength training and flexibility activities.

Here are some focused activities that help strengthen your stomach and improve your digestive health:

• **Core exercises:** These are workouts that target the abdominal and lower back muscles, which are critical for supporting your spine and internal organs.

Core exercises can also help you shed belly fat, which lowers inflammation and improves your gut microbiota. Core exercises include planks, crunches, and leg raises.

• **Low-impact activities**: These are activities that do not place undue strain on your joints, such as walking, swimming, cycling, or yoga. Low-impact activities can benefit your cardiovascular health by increasing blood circulation and oxygen delivery to your intestines.

They can also help you relax and reduce stress, which can benefit both your gut health and mood. Low-impact activities include walking, swimming, cycling, and yoga.

• **Yoga poses**: These are physical positions that you hold while breathing deeply and focusing your thoughts. Yoga positions can target several regions of the body, including the belly.

Some yoga poses can aid with digestion, reduce gas and bloating, and detoxify the body. Yoga poses that are healthy for your gut include cat-cow pose, child's pose, and wind-relieving pose.

These are some of the workouts that might help strengthen your gut and improve your health. Remember to check with your doctor before beginning any new fitness regimen, especially if you have any medical concerns or injuries.

Remember to drink plenty of water, eat a balanced diet, and take probiotics to improve your gut health. Have fun exercising!

CONCLUSION

Thank you for reading this book about gut health diets. I hope you've learned a lot about how your gut influences your health and well-being, and how you can enhance it by eating a healthy diet, taking probiotics, and exercising often.

Your gut not only digests the food you eat, but it also houses trillions of microorganisms that affect your immunity, mood, metabolism, and other functions. A healthy gut can help you prevent or manage a variety of chronic illnesses, including diabetes, obesity, heart disease, and cancer. A healthy stomach can also improve your mood, energy, and confidence.

In this book, I've included a complete and structured shopping list, a two-week meal plan, and a range of gut-friendly, healthy recipes. I've also provided you with some advice and suggestions for gut-friendly exercise, as well as examples of specialized activities that help strengthen your gut and improve your digestive health.

However, this book is not intended to replace the advice of your doctor or other health care provider. Everyone's intuition is unique, so what works for one person may not work for another.

As a result, before beginning any new diet or fitness regimen, visit your doctor, particularly if you have any medical issues or sensitivities. Your doctor can help you tailor your gut health diet to your specific needs and goals.

I hope you enjoyed this book and found it useful and enlightening. If you did, please provide positive feedback and share it with your friends and family. Your feedback and support are greatly welcomed, and they will help me develop future works.

I appreciate your time and attention. I wish you all the best for your gut health and overall well-being. Have a good day.

www.ingramcontent.com/pod-product-compliance
Lightning Source LLC
Chambersburg PA
CBHW070759260726
48660CB00005B/1687